Ketogenic Diet

Nutritious Low Card Meals That Burn Fat Fast

©Abel Jones

Table of Contents

Introduction

The burning sensation in your chest after climbing up two flights of stairs, jeans that don't fit, and friends that tell you "I think you're getting fat,"— are you tired of all these? Are you in dire need of losing weight and practically burning all the excess fat you have in your body?

Right now, maybe you're feeling awful about your weight and physical appearance, but let me tell you this: the moment that you decided that you need to do something about your dilemma (like purchasing this book), means you're already halfway to losing weight, improving your health, and becoming a better version of you.

But before I introduce this effective and revolutionary diet that will help solve your problems, let's straighten up things first. Let me ask you these questions:

What is the real reason why you want to shed fat and lose weight? Is it to boost your confidence and have a perfect bikini body?

You see, there's nothing wrong about wanting to lose weight in order to become more attractive, but that shouldn't be your main focus. Besides achieving a "desirable" body, your main purpose of going on a diet should be to become healthy and avoid the complications of being overweight or obese.

The World Health Organization (WHO) defines overweight and obesity as an "abnormal or excessive fat accumulation that may impair health." Experts have recognized that the primary cause of these conditions are a deadly combination of an unhealthy diet, plus a sedentary lifestyle.

It is quite disturbing to note that over 1.9 billion adults all over the world are suffering these conditions (WHO,

2014); 42 million children below 5 years old are also either obese or overweight.

Now you might be asking why you should care about the effects of these conditions other than becoming physically attractive. Well, that's because carrying extra pounds in your body puts you at great risk of developing chronic illnesses such as: stroke, heart disease, type 2 diabetes, osteoarthritis, breast cancer, colon cancer, to name a few. Although these complications may alarm you, the good news is that obesity and overweight can be reversed and the complications that go with it are preventable; and I'm sure you already know the answer how—a healthy diet!

Maybe you've already tried some of the fad diets that are popular right now, but they seem to not work. Or probably you have also tried some of the fasting and starvation diets out there that promises instant results, but you just can't seem to keep up with the idea of skipping meals. Well, maybe it's time that you try a diet that is scientifically proven to help you burn fat, lose weight, and provide you other health benefits—the Ketogenic Diet.

Also called as the Keto Diet, this food program is a low carb-high fat diet that "forces" the body to enter into a different metabolic state where fat is burned as fuel for energy instead of glucose (I will discuss this further later).

You may think that the Keto Diet is a fairly new food regimen and is also a fad, but on the contrary, this diet has already became popular in the 1940's when it was used to help minimize seizures of children with epilepsy.

However, it lost its place under the spotlight when anticonvulsant drugs became available to the market. It only gained popularity again in the 1990's when a son of a Hollywood director who had epilepsy underwent the diet which helped him reduce his epileptic episodes.

This paved way for further research on the Keto Diet. These studies found that this low carb-high fat diet was not only able to help minimize seizures for patients with epilepsy, but it can also help individuals to lose weight, minimize abdominal fat, increase HDL and LDL levels (good cholesterol), decrease blood sugar levels, prevent cancer and cognitive decline. So in short, this diet that I'm about to introduce to you will not only help you burn fat and lose weight, but it can also deliver other amazing benefits for your over-all health!

Before I go any further, I'd like to thank and congratulate you for purchasing this book, "Ketogenic Diet: Low Carb Meals that Burn Fat Fast".

This book will help you learn and understand what the Ketogenic Diet is and how you can use this to lose weight—fast! The chapters of this book will provide you with the information on how you can start transitioning in a ketosis state, how you can create your own Keto meal plan, and I will also provide you a comprehensive list of Ketogenic Diet approved foods. Of course, I've also included delicious Keto recipes for breakfast, lunch, and dinner, and most importantly, a month Keto eating plan that can help guide you on your first month in the Keto Diet.

Today is a beginning of a better and healthier you.

Chapter 1

How to Get Started: Transitioning Into Ketosis

You've heard of countless low-carb diets that help you lose weight and at the same time deliver amazing health benefits, but a low carb-high fat diet? *How does that work? How can eating more fat, help you lose fat?* Well, that is what where the metabolic processes *ketosis* steps in to help.

The "Normal" Diet vs. Keto Diet

Ever since modern agriculture was introduced, man's normal diet has shifted from being meat and vegetable eaters (our hunter and gatherer ancestors) to individuals who eat more processed carbohydrates such as pasta, bread, rice and potatoes.

Now, there's nothing wrong with carbs. Carbs per se isn't actually bad for our health as long as we consume more of the healthy types of carbs such as vegetables (yes they contain carbs too), legumes, whole-grains, fruits, and nuts.

However, if you really want to lose weight and also prevent developing type 2 diabetes, then it would be advisable to limit the amount of carbs you consume. That's because when you eat foods high in carbohydrates they get broken down in your blood as glucose (sugar). This means that when you consume lots of carbs, a high amount of glucose becomes present in your blood, therefore resulting in high blood sugar levels.

Again, carbs aren't all bad because in a normal diet the body will reach out for glucose in order to use it as fuel for energy, as well as fuel the other functions of our body. The only problem is that any glucose that isn't used by the body as energy will be stored as body fat.

This is one of the main reasons why a lot of people in today's day and age are overweight, because they consume to many carbs and only expend little of it due to their sedentary lifestyle.

The Ketogenic Diet on the other hand reduces the consumption of carbs to a minimal and increases healthy fats in one's diet. When carbs are reduced, your body will naturally look for other sources to burn for energy and in this case, fats are chosen. The Ketogenic Diet shifts your body into a metabolic state called ketosis, a process that burns fat instead of glucose allowing you to shed unwanted weight easily and quickly.

Entering into Ketosis

As you now know, the target of the Ketogenic Diet is to allow your body to enter into ketosis; but the question now is, how?

There are three different types of Ketogenic Diets— the Standard Ketogenic Diet (SKD), Cyclical Ketogenic Diet (CKD), and the Targeted Ketogenic Diet (TKD). People who have sedentary lifestyles and wish to lose weight through this diet is advised to follow the SKD. This diet recommends to limit the consumption of your carbs to 20-50 grams daily, which means your macros should be made up of 70%-75% fat, 20%-25% protein, and 5%-10% carbs. The number of daily calories you can consume however, relies on your weight, height, age, and activity. If you're unsure how to do this, you can always consult a keto calculator (click here).

You might be a little skeptical about the Ketogenic Diet right now, especially if you think that you need to only consume small amount of carbs in your diet. But if you consume a healthy number of calories and eat foods that are nutrient dense (ex. vegetables, and healthy fat), then you don't have to worry about going hungry at all! You can safely enter into a state of ketosis when you do this.

However, I'd like to remind you that unlike any other diets, the Keto Diet needs your complete commitment to the diet in order for you to achieve the state of ketosis. Depending on your body type, activity level, and your diet, you can get into ketosis anywhere from 2 days to a week. For beginners, it is advisable that you use urine ketone sticks (such as Ketostix) to monitor the levels of ketones in your body and ensure that you are in ketosis state. This is a useful tip to help you know whether your body is under ketosis and is burning fat as energy.

I must advise you however, that before anything else, it is a must that you ask for a green light from your health care provider if you are planning to follow the Ketogenic Diet; or any type of diet. Although this diet is over-all safe, even for kids, you have to let your doctor know about this especially if you have existing health conditions.

Pregnant women or those who are breastfeeding aren't encouraged to try the Ketogenic Diet for weight loss because this may have adverse effects on their baby.

Chapter 2

Ketogenic Diet Food List

Time to purge your pantry and replace them with these Ketogenic Diet approved foods!

Fats and Oils

Since fat will make the majority of your meals, it is a must that you choose the good type (natural sources) of fat and not those that are dangerous to your health. Some of your best choices for fat are:

Ghee or Clarified butter

Avocado

Coconut Oil

Red Palm Oil

Butter

Coconut Butter

Peanut Butter

Chicken Fat

Beef Tallow

Non-hydrogenated Lard

Macadamia Nuts

Egg Yolks

Fish rich in Omega-3 Fatty Acids like salmon, mackerel, trout, tuna, and even shell fish.

Protein

In order to achieve a state of ketosis, you need to consume 20%-25% protein in your daily caloric allowance. This means your consumption of fat will be high, carbs are low, and protein, moderate. Of course, you also want to choose the healthy sources of protein that are either organic, or grass fed.

Meat— beef, veal, lamb, chicken, duck, pheasant, pork chops, pork loin, etc.

Deli Meat— bacon, sausage, ham (make sure to watch out of added sugar and other fillers)

Eggs— preferably free-range or organic eggs

Fish— wild caught salmon, catfish, halibut, trout, tuna, etc.

Seafood— lobster, crab, oyster, clams, mussels

Peanut Butter—this is a great source of protein, but make sure to choose the all-natural variant

Dairy

Compared to other weight loss diets, in the Ketogenic Diet, you are encouraged to choose dairy products that are full fat. Some of the best dairy products that you can choose are:

Hard and Soft Cheese— cream cheese, mozzarella, cheddar, etc.

Cottage Cheese

Heavy Whipping Cream

Sour Cream

Full-Fat Yogurt

Vegetables

Over-all, vegetables are rich in vitamins and minerals that contribute to a healthy body. However, if you're aiming to avoid carbs, it's best that you keep away from starchy vegetables such as potatoes, yam, peas, corn, beans, and legumes. You also want to limit vegetables that taste sweet such as carrots and squash. Instead, stick with green leafy vegetables that are preferably organically grown and other low-carb veggies.

Spinach	Alfalfa Sprouts
Lettuce	Celery
Collard Greens	Tomato
Mustard Greens	*Broccoli
Bok Choi	*Cauliflower
Kale	*eat occasionally

Fruits

You choice of fruit is only limited to avocado and some *berries because fruits are high in carbs and sugar.

Drinks

Water

Black Coffee

Herbal Tea

Wine—white wine and dry red wine are OK, as long as they are only consumed occasionally

Others

Homemade Mayo—if you want to buy mayo from the store, make sure that you watch out for the carbs it contains

Homemade Mustard

Any type of Spices and Herbs

*Honey

*Stevia

*Agave Nectar

*Catsup (Sugar-free)

*Dark Chocolate/Cocoa

Food List by Colour

Green List

This is an all-you-can-eat list - you choose anything you like without worrying about the carbohydrate content as all the foods will be between 0 to 5g/100g.

It will be almost impossible to overdo your carbohydrate intake by sticking to this group of foods. Overeating protein is not recommended, so eat a moderate amount of animal protein at each meal. Include as much fat as you are comfortable with - bearing in mind that Keto is high in fat. Caution: even though these are all-you-can-eat foods, only eat when hungry, stop when full and do not overeat. The size and thickness of your palm without fingers is a good measure for a serving of animal protein. All meat, eggs, dairy and greens should be organic, free range and grass fed where possible.

ANIMAL PROTEIN

(unless these have a rating, they are all 0g/100g)

All eggs

All meats, poultry and game

All natural and cured meats (pancetta, parma ham, coppa etc)

All natural and cured sausages (salami, chorizo etc)

All offal

All seafood (except swordfish and tilefish - high mercury content)

Broths

DAIRY

Cottage cheese

Cream

Cream cheese

Full-cream Greek yoghurt

Full-cream milk

Hard cheeses

Soft cheeses

FATS

Any rendered animal fat

Avocado oil

Butter

Cheese - firm, natural, full-fat, aged cheeses (not processed)

Coconut oil

Duck fat

Ghee

Lard

Macadamia oil

Mayonnaise, full fat only (not from seeds oils)

Olive oil

FLAVOURINGS AND CONDIMENTS

All flavourings and condiments are okay, provided they do not contain sugars and preservatives or vegetable (seed) oils.

NUTS AND SEEDS

Almonds

Flaxseeds (watch out for pre-ground flaxseeds, they go rancid quickly and become toxic)

Macadamia nuts

Pecan nuts

Pine nuts

Pumpkin seeds

Sunflower seeds

Walnuts

SWEETENERS

Erythritol granules

Stevia powder

Xylitol granules

VEGETABLES

All green leafy vegetables (spinach, cabbage, lettuces etc)

Any other vegetables grown above the ground (except butternut)

Artichoke hearts

Asparagus

Aubergines

Avocados

Broccoli

Brussel sprouts

Cabbage

Cauliflower

Celery

Courgettes

Leeks

Mushrooms

Olives

Onions

Peppers

Pumpkin

Radishes

Sauerkraut

Spring onions

Tomatoes

Orange List

Chart your carbohydrates without getting obsessive and still obtain an excellent outcome. If you are endeavouring to go into ketosis, this list will assist you to stay under a total of 50g carbs for the day. These are all net carbs and they are all 23 to 25g per indicated amount. Ingredients are all fresh unless otherwise indicated.

FRUITS

Apples 1.5

Bananas 1 small

Blackberries 3.5 C

Blueberries 1.5 C

Cherries (sweet) 1 C

Clementines 3

Figs 3 small

Gooseberries 1.5 C

Grapes (green) under 1 C

Guavas 2

Kiwi fruits 3

Litchis 18

Mangos, sliced, under 1 C

Nectarines 2

Oranges 2

Pawpaw 1

Peaches 2

Pears (Bartlett) 1

Pineapple, sliced, 1 C

Plums 4

Pomegranate ½

Prickly pears 4

Quinces 2

Raspberries 2 C

Strawberries 25

Watermelon 2 C

NUTS

Cashews, raw, 6 T

Chestnuts, raw, 1 C

SWEETENERS

Honey 1 t

VEGETABLES

Butternut 1.5 C

Carrots 5

Sweet potato 0.5 C

KEY

C	=	cups	per	day
T	=	tablespoons	per	day
t	=	teaspoons	per	day
g	=	grams	per	day

For example: 1.5 apples are all the carbs you can have off the orange list for the day (if you want to go into ketosis and make sure you are under 50g total carbs for the day).

Red List

Red will contain all the foods to avoid as they will be either toxic (e.g. seed oils, soya) or high-carbohydrate foods (e.g. potatoes, rice).

We strongly suggest you avoid all the items on this list, or, at best, eat them very occasionally and restrict the amount when you do. They will do nothing to help you in your attempt to reach your goal.

BAKED GOODS

All flours from grains - wheat flour, cornflour, rye flour, barley flour, pea flour, rice flour etc

All forms of bread

All grains - wheat, oats, barley, rye, amaranth, quinoa, teff etc

Beans (dried)

"Breaded" or battered foods

Brans

Breakfast cereals, muesli, granola of any kind

Buckwheat

Cakes, biscuits, confectionary

Corn products - popcorn, polenta, corn thins, maize

Couscous

Crackers, cracker breads

Millet

Pastas, noodles

Rice

Rice cakes

Sorghum

Spelt

Thickening agents such as gravy powder, maize starch or stock cubes

BEVERAGES

Beer, cider

Fizzy drinks (sodas) of any description other than carbonated water

Lite, zero, diet drinks of any description

DAIRY / DAIRY-RELATED

Cheese spreads, commercial spreads

Coffee creamers

Commercial almond milk

Condensed milk

Fat-free anything

Ice cream

Puddings

Reduced-fat cow's milk

Rice milk

Soy milk

FATS

All seed oils (safflower, sunflower, canola, grapeseed, cottonseed, corn)

Chocolate

Commercial sauces, marinades and salad dressings

Hydrogenated or partially hydrogenated oils including margarine, vegetable oils, vegetable fats

Ketogenic Diet Foods and their Macros

Protein Source				
	Fats (g)	Net Carbs (g)	Protein (g)	Calories
1 oz. beef sirloin (broiled)	4	0	7.7	69
1 oz. ground beef, 30% fat (broiled)	5.1	0	7.1	77
1 oz. chicken, white meat	1.3	0	8.8	49
1 egg (large)	4.8	0.4	6.3	72
1 slice bacon (baked)	3.5	0	2.9	44
1 oz. smoked ham	2.6	0	6.4	50
1 oz. beef hotdog	8.5	0.5	3.1	92
1 oz. pork chop (broiled)	4.1	0	6.7	65
1 oz. pork ribs (roasted)	8.3	0	6.2	102
1 oz. lamb chop (broiled)	3.9	0	7.3	67
1 oz. tuna (cooked)	1.8	0	8.5	52
1 oz. salmon (raw)	1.8	0	5.6	40
1 oz. shrimp (cooked)	0.1	0	6.8	28

Vegetables

	Fats (g)	Net Carbs (g)	Protein (g)	Calories
1 oz. spinach (raw)	0.1	0.4	0.8	7
1 oz. romaine lettuce	0.1	0.3	0.4	5
1 oz. broccoli (cooked)	0.1	1.1	0.7	10
1 oz. cauliflower (cooked	0.1	0.5	0.5	7
1 oz. celery (raw)	0	0.3	0.7	5
1 oz. cucumber (raw)	0	1	0.2	4
1 oz. green beans (cooked)	0.1	1.3	0.5	10
1 oz. snow peas (cooked)	0	2.8	1.5	24
1 oz. tomato (raw)	0	0.8	0.3	5
1 oz. butternut squash (baked)	0	2.1	0.3	11
1 oz. green bell pepper	0	0.8	0.2	6
1 clove of garlic	0	1	0.2	4
1 oz. white onion (raw)	0	2.1	0.3	11
1 oz. green onion (raw)	0	1.3	0.5	9

	Fats (g)	Net Carbs (g)	Protein (g)	Calories
1 oz. avocado	4.4	0.6	0.6	47
1 oz. button mushrooms (raw)	0.2	0.6	0.9	6

Dairy Products

	Fats (g)	Net Carbs (g)	Protein (g)	Calories
1 oz. whole milk	1	1.5	1	19
1 oz. heavy cream	11	0.8	0.6	103
1 oz. half and half cream	3.5	1.3	0.9	39
1 oz. full-fat sour cream	5.6	0.8	0.6	55
1 oz. whole buttermilk	0.9	1.4	0.9	18
1 oz. cheddar cheese	9.4	0.4	7.1	114
1 oz. whole-milk mozzarella	6.3	0.6	6.3	85
1 oz. parmesan	7.3	0.9	10.1	111
1 oz. Swiss cheese	7.9	1.5	7.6	108
1 oz. mascarpone	13	1	1	130
1 oz. cream cheese	9.7	1.1	1.7	97
1 oz. feta cheese	6	1.2	4	75

Nuts and Seeds

	Fats (g)	Net Carbs (g)	Protein (g)	Calories

1 oz. almonds (raw)	15	3	6	170
1 oz. cashew nuts (raw)	13	7	5	160
1 oz. hazelnuts (raw)	17	2	4	176
1 oz. walnuts (raw)	18	2	4	185
1 oz. pistachios (raw)	13	5	6	158
1 oz. pumpkin seeds (raw)	14	1	8	159
1 oz. flax seeds (raw)	10	0	7	131
1 oz. chia seeds (raw)	100	0	7	160
1 oz. sesame seeds (raw)	14	4	5	160

Chapter 3

Creating Your Own Meal Plan

Remember that in order to lose weight in the Ketogenic Diet, you have to let your body enter into the metabolic state of ketosis. Without this, your body will still continue to burn glucose as fuel and would store as fat any excess sugar that isn't used as fuel. In order for you to enter into ketosis, you have to decrease your consumption of carbs, increase your intake of fat, and moderately eat protein.

As you know, the foods you eat are key to reset your body into a different metabolic state, that's why it is very important that you create your own meal plan so that you are sure that everything you eat will not disrupt your metabolism's state of ketosis. My advice is that you *determine the macros that you need to consume through the use of this keto calculator* so that you can achieve weight loss through the diet.

After you have identified the number of grams of macros that you should consume daily for your body type, stick with this number when you create your meal plan.

For example, John, who is an average 6-foot tall male who weighs 190 lbs. (86.2 kg) and lives a sedentary lifestyle. According to the keto calculator, in order for John to lose weight and enter ketosis, he must maintain a daily diet of 1654 kcal made with 25g carbs (6%), 91g protein (22%), and 132g fat (72%).

With these numbers— 1654 calories, 25g net carbs, 91g protein, and 132g fat, John should create a meal plan to help him achieve this.

I've provided you with a meal plan in the last chapter of this book that you can use in the early weeks of your Ketogenic Diet, or you can also create a meal plan of your own with these following tips:

Helpful Tips for the Ketogenic Diet

Learn to Count Your Net Carbs— As you now know, the key to entering a state of ketosis is to limit your carbs to 20-25grams (net carbs) every day. One of the useful tools to help you monitor this is through the use of an app called MyFitnessPal (I encourage you to download this on your device!). With this app, you can easily log your foods which can help you monitor the foods you consume.

Although this app doesn't provide you with your consumption of net carbs, but it will provide you with the fiber and carbs that you have consumed. To get your net carbs, just simply subtract the fiber from the carbs you consumed.

Beware of Hidden Carbs— It will be very easy for you to avoid foods such as pastas and bread because you know that they contain loads of carbs. However, what most people fail to do is to also count the carbs that are "hidden" in foods such as baked beans, salad dressing, and tomato sauce which all have carbs in them! So make sure to read labels and count all carbs to stick to the 20-25 grams daily and achieve ketosis.

Choose the Right Foods— Even if the Ketogenic Diet is a low carb-high fat diet, this doesn't give you the liberty to consume as much fat as you can. Of course you want the food you consume to be of quality and are rich in nutrients. But one good tip to remember is to just stay away from carbs such as pastas, breads, rice, and even sugar. The 20-25 grams of carbs that you're allowed to consume should be made of vegetables that also have carbs in them.

Limit Your Consumption of Fruit— We all know that fruits have loads of vitamins, fiber, and other nutrients that are good for the body. However, if you want to reset your metabolism and allow it to use fat as fuel instead of glucose, then you must limit your consumption of fruit to a minimum. That's because all fruits are high in fructose (a type of sugar found in fruit), which causes your insulin levels to spike. When that happens, the fats cells in your body are locked and your body will use glucose as energy.

Remember that in the Ketogenic Diet, you are only allowed to have 20-25 grams of net carbs a day. A medium-sized banana already amounts to 24g net carbs, which means, you almost have already consumed all your carbs for the day in just eating a banana. If you still want to consume fruits, you can stick with a cup of mixed berries that has 5g net carbs, but this is not recommended to be consumed daily.

Spend More Time in the Kitchen— For you to achieve ketosis, it is vital that you watch over the foods you eat. That's why it is advisable if you prepare your own meals and avoid eating out too much. Yes, you will have to sacrifice a bit of your time in preparing your meals, but this assures you that you're only consuming what is approved in the Ketogenic Diet.

I've provided you with a list of recipes from breakfast to dinner in the next chapters to help you whip up your own Keto-approved meals in your kitchen; turn to the next chapter now!

Chapter 4

Easy Ketogenic Diet Breakfast

Breakfast Granola

Ingredients

½ cup almonds

½ cup walnuts

½ cup hazelnuts, chopped

½ cup coconut flakes

½ cup mixed seeds (pumpkin seeds, flaxseeds, sunflower seeds, etc.)

2 tsp. cinnamon, ground

3 tbsp. coconut oil, melted

Directions

1. Preheat oven at 350F
2. Combine all the ingredients in a large bowl and stir well.
3. Transfer the mixture in a baking tray and place in the oven to cook for about 20 minutes. Shake every 5 minutes to make sure that the granola doesn't burn.
4. Let it cook and store in an airtight container.
5. Consume with a bowl of full-cream yogurt.

Nutritional Info (1/2 cup)

Calories: 210

Net Carbs: 30g

Fat: 8g

Protein: 6g

Buttermilk Seed Rusks

Ingredients

½ cup butter, melted

1 cup buttermilk

4 eggs

1 cup almond flour

1 cup ground flax

2 cups desiccated coconut

1 cup mixed seeds

2 ½ tsp. baking powder

1 tsp. salt

½ cup Xylitol

Directions

1. Preheat oven at 350F
2. In a bowl, combine the yogurt, butter, and eggs.
3. Slowly add the dry ingredients and stir well to make a batter.
4. Carefully transfer the mixture into a baking tray and cook in the oven for 45 minutes.
5. Allow to cool down before slicing it into 30 rusk shapes.
6. Place on a wire rack upside down, and cook in the oven again for 90 minutes at 210F.

Nutritional Info (1 rusk)

Calories: 119

Net Carbs: 17g

Fat: 3g

Protein: 2g

Caprese Stack

Ingredients

3 slices mozzarella cheese

2 large slices of tomato

4 fresh basil leaves

salt and pepper

1 tsp. olive oil

Directions

1. On a plate, stack the mozzarella cheese, tomato, and basil.
2. Season with salt and pepper and drizzle with olive oil

Nutritional Info (per stack)

Calories:186

Net Carbs: 5g

Fat: 10g

Protein: 6g

34

Breakfast Quiche

Ingredients

3 tbsp. coconut oil

5 whole eggs

8 slices of bacon, cooked and chopped

100ml cream

2 cups baby spinach, roughly chopped

1 cup red pepper, chopped

1 cup green pepper, chopped

1 cup yellow onion, chopped

2 cloves of garlic, minced

1 cup mushrooms, chopped

100g cheddar cheese, grated

salt to taste

Directions

1. Preheat oven at 375F
2. In a large bowl, mix all vegetables including the mushrooms together.
3. In another small bowl, whisk the 5 eggs with the cream
4. Carefully scoop the veggie mixture into a muffin pan coated with cooking spray, top with egg and cheese filling up to ¾ of the muffin tins. Sprinkle with chopped bacon on top.
5. Place in the oven to bake for 15 minutes or until the top of the quiche are firm.

6. Let it cook for a few minutes before serving.

Nutritional Info (1 small quiche)

Calories: 210

Net Carbs: 5g

Fat: 13g

Protein: 6g

Easy Pancakes

Ingredients

1 tbsp. melted butter

2 eggs

5 tbsp. full-fat milk

1 tbsp. xylitol

½ tsp salt

2 tbsp. coconut flour

1 tbsp. almond flour

½ tsp. baking powder

Directions

1. In a bowl, whisk the eggs with the milk, salt, xylitol, and melted butter (room temp.)
2. Add the coconut and almond flour to the mixture, along with the baking powder. Mix well.
3. Heat a non-stick pan over medium fire and scoop 3 tbsp. of the batter to make pancakes.
4. Flip the pancake when bubbles start to form and cook until golden brown.
5. Serve with ½ cup of berries on the side.

Nutritional Info (1 pc.)

Calories: 194

Net Carbs: 30g

Fat: 13g

Protein: 31g

Ketogenic Mug Bread

Ingredients

1 tbsp. coconut flour

3 tbsp. almond flour

1 tsp. baking powder

1 whole egg

1 tsp. melted butter

3 tbsp. water

a pinch of salt

Directions

1. Add all the dry ingredients in a bowl then add the egg and water and mix well make sure there are no lumps in your mixture.
2. Pour the melted butter in the cup you are going to use. You can also use the cup to melt the butter to begin with, but make sure not to over heat the butter, 5 seconds in the microwave should be more than enough. Now swirl the butter around the cup make sure to coat the inside of the cup then pour the butter into the bread mix and combine.
3. Pour the mix in your cup and microwave for 1.5 mins. if you are planning on doubling the mix I would suggest using a bigger wider mug or the mix will not cook all the way through. Don't microwave for more than 3 min or the mix will end up hard.
4. Once you have removed it from the mug, you can then slice it into rounds and place it in the toaster to crisp it up a little.

Nutritional Info (1 serving)

Calories: 238

Net Carbs: 2.6g

Fat: 19g

Protein: 13g

Veggie Scramble

Ingredients

4 egg whites

1 egg yolk

2 tbsp. almond milk

1 cup spinach

1 tomato, chopped

½ white onion, chopped

3 fresh basil leaves, chopped

salt and pepper to taste

ghee

Directions

1. In a bowl, whisk the egg yolk and whites with the milk. Stir well.
2. Heat the ghee on a pan over medium heat. Add the onions and sauté until fragrant.
3. Throw in the tomato to the pan with the spinach and cook until the spinach is almost wilted.
4. Pour the egg mixture to the spinach and cook until firm or until the egg sets. Stir constantly.
5. Season with salt and pepper.
6. Serve warm

Nutritional Info (per serving)

Calories: 203

Net Carbs: 18g

Fat: 5g

Protein: 20g

Egg Pesto Scramble

Ingredients

3 eggs

1 tbsp. pesto sauce

1 tbsp. olive oil

2 tbsp. sour cream

Directions

1. Whisk the eggs in a bowl and season with salt and pepper.
2. Heat a non-stick pan over low heat. Drizzle with olive oil and pour the eggs. Constantly whisk the eggs while cooking.
3. Add the pesto mixture to the eggs and stir well.
4. Turn off the fire and mix in the sour cream. Combine well.
5. Serve with 1/2 cup mashed avocado.

Nutritional Info (per serving)

Calories: 467

Net Carbs: 3.3g

Fat: 41.5g

Protein: 20.4g

Cheesy Keto Bread

Ingredients

125g full-fat cream cheese

1 cup cheddar cheese, grated

3 large eggs

1 tsp. apple cider vinegar

2 cups almond flour

2 tsp. baking powder

1 tsp. mustard powder

1 tsp. salt

Directions

1. Preheat oven at 375F
2. Combine all the ingredients in a bowl with a hand mixer, except the cheddar cheese.
3. Add the cheddar cheese to the mixture and combine using a spatula or a fork. Be careful not to mush the cheese.
4. Line a bread tin with well-greased baking paper and bake in the oven for 45 minutes.

Nutritional Info (per serving)

Calories:495

Net Carbs: 6.5g

Fat: 9.6g

Protein: 19.7g

46

Lemon Cheesecake Breakfast Mousse

Ingredients

3 tbsp. cream cheese

1 tbsp. lemon juice

50ml heavy cream (look for those with zero carbs)

100ml Yoghurt

1tbsp. Xylitol

1/8 tsp. salt

2 tbsp. whey protein

Directions

1. Blend cream cheese and lemon juice in a bowl until smooth.
2. Add heavy cream and blend until whipped. Gently add in yoghurt.
3. Taste and adjust sweetener if needed.
4. Serve with ¼ cup berry coulis.

Berry Breakfast Shake

Ingredients

¾ cup mixed berries

1 cup almond milk

1 tbsp. all-natural peanut butter

1 tbsp. protein powder

¼ tsp. cinnamon powder

¼ tsp. ginger, minced

Directions

1. Place all the ingredients in a blender and mix until smooth.

Nutritional Info (per serving)

Calories: 319

Net Carbs: 9g

Fat: 15g

Protein: 28g

Cacao and Raspberry Pudding

Ingredients

1 tbsp. cacao powder

¼ cup raspberry

3 tbsp. chia seeds

1 cup almond milk

1 tsp. agave

Directions

2. In a small bowl, combine the almond milk and cacao powder. Stir well.
3. Add the chia seeds to the bowl and let it rest for 5 minutes.
4. Using a fork, fluff the chia and cacao mixture and then place in the fridge to chill for at least 30 minutes.
5. Serve with raspberries and a drizzle of agave on top

Coco and Blueberry Smoothie

Serves 2

Ingredients

½ cup blueberries

½ cup coconut cream

1 tbsp. coconut oil

½ cup almond milk, vanilla flavor

3 ice cubes

Directions

1. Place all the ingredients in a blender and mix until you achieve a smooth consistency.

Creamy Chocolate Milk

Serves 2

Ingredients.

16 ounces unsweetened almond milk

1 teaspoon xylitol

4 ounces heavy cream

1 scoop Whey Chocolate Isolate powder

1/2 cup crushed ice (optional: add if you like a thick drink, but the flavor will be less intense.)

Directions

1. Put all ingredients in blender and blend until smooth.
2. This recipe can be doubled, as can most low carb smoothie recipes.

Nutrition info for one serving:

292 calories,

25 grams of fat,

15 grams of protein,

4 carbs.

Blueberry Almond Smoothie

Serves 2

Ingredients

16 ounces unsweetened almond milk

1 teaspoon xylitol

4 ounces heavy cream

1/4 cup frozen unsweetened blueberries

1 scoop Whey Vanilla protein powder

Directions

1. Put all ingredients in blender and blend until smooth.
2. Add a little water if it becomes too thick.
3. Measure those blueberries as they add more carbs.

Nutrition info for one serving:

302 calories,

25 grams of fat,

15 grams of protein,

6 grams carbs,

1 grams fiber.

Mozzarella, Red Pepper & Bacon Frittata

Serves 6

Ingredients

Olive oil (1 tablespoon)

Parsley (2 tablespoons, chopped)

Mozzarella cheese (4 oz., cubed)

Bell pepper (1, red, chopped)

Heavy cream (1/4 cup)

Salt

Bacon (7 slices)

Bella mushrooms (4 caps, large)

Basil (1/2 cup, chopped)

Goat cheese (2 oz., grated)

Eggs (9)

Parmesan cheese (1/4 cup, grated)

Black pepper

Directions

1. Set oven to 350 F.
2. Chop red pepper, bacon, basil and mushroom. Slice mozzarella into cubes and put aside.
3. Heat olive oil in a skillet until it slightly smokes then add bacon and cook for 5 minutes until browned.

54

4. Add red pepper and cook for 2 minutes until soft. While pepper cooks, add cream, parmesan cheese, eggs and black pepper to a bowl and whisk to combine.
5. Add mushrooms to pot, stir and cook for 5 minutes until soaked in fat. Add basil, cook for 1 minute then add mozzarella.
6. Put in egg mixture and use spoon to move ingredients around so that the egg gets on the bottom of pan.
7. Top with goat cheese and place in oven for 8 minutes then broil for 6 minutes.
8. Use knife to pry frittata edges from pan and place on a plate and slice.
9. Serve.

Nutritional Information

Calories 408

Net Carbs 2.4g

Fats 31.2g

Protein 19.2g

Fiber 0.8g

Rosemary, Sausage & Cheese Pies

Serves 2

Ingredients

Cheddar cheese (3/4 cup, grated)

Coconut oil (1/4 cup)

Egg yolks (5)

Rosemary (1/2 teaspoon)

Baking soda (1/4 teaspoon)

Chicken sausage (1 ½)

Coconut flour (1/4 cup)

Coconut milk (2 tablespoons)

Lemon juice (2 teaspoons)

Cayenne pepper (1/4 teaspoon)

Kosher salt (1/8 teaspoon)

Directions

1. Set oven to 350 F.
2. Chop sausage, heat skillet and cook sausage. While sausages cook combine all dry ingredients in a bowl. In another bowl combine lemon juice, oil and coconut milk. Add liquids to dry mixture and add ½ cup of cheese; fold to combine and put into 2 ramekins.
3. Add cooked sausages to batter and use spoon to push into mixture.
4. Bake for 25 minutes until golden on top. Top with leftover cheese and broil for 4 minutes.

5. Serve warm.

Nutritional Information

Calories 711

Net Carbs 5.8g

Fats 65.3g

Protein 34.3g

Fiber 11.5g

Chia, Coconut & Almond Oatmeal

Serves 2

Ingredients

Chia seeds (1/4 cup)

Coconut flakes (1/3 cup, unsweetened)

Vanilla (1 teaspoon, sugar free)

Almond milk (1 cup, unsweetened)

Stevia extract (10 drops)

Coconut (1/4 cup, shredded, unsweetened)

Almonds (1/3 cup, flaked)

Heavy whipping cream (1/2 cup)

Erythritol (2 tablespoons)

Directions

1. Place almond and coconut flakes in a pot and toast for 3 minutes until fragrant.
2. Place toasted ingredients into a bowl along with chia seeds, erythritol and shredded coconut; mix together to combine.
3. Top with milk and stir. You can use hot or cold milk based on your preference.
4. Add vanilla and stevia, stir and set aside for 5-10 minutes.
5. Serve. May be topped with fresh berries.

Nutritional Information

Calories 359

Net Carbs 5g

Fats 30.4g

Protein 9.4 g

Fiber 10.5g

Breakfast Berry Shake

Serves 3

Ingredients

Mixed berries (3/4 cup)

Almond milk (1 cup)

All-natural peanut butter (1 tablespoon)

Protein powder (1 tablespoon)

Cinnamon powder (1/4 teaspoons)

Ginger, minced (1/4 teaspoons)

Directions

1. Place all the ingredients in a blender and mix until smooth.

Nutritional Information

Calories: 319

Net Carbs: 9g

Fat: 15g

Protein: 28g

Breakfast Cheese Tacos

Serves 3

Ingredients

Eggs (6)

Bacon (3 strips)

Cheddar cheese (1 oz., shredded)

Mozzarella cheese (1 cup, shredded)

Butter (2 tablespoons)

Avocado (1/2, cubed)

Salt

Black pepper

Directions

1. Cook bacon until crisp, put aside until needed.
2. Heat a non-stick pan and place 1/3 cup mozzarella into pan and cook for 3 minutes until browned around the edges. Place a wooden spoon across a bowl or pot and use tongs to lift cheese 'taco from pot. Repeat with leftover cheese.
3. Melt butter in a skillet and scramble eggs; use pepper and salt to season.
4. Spoon eggs into hardened shells and top with avocado and bacon.
5. Top with cheddar and serve.

Nutritional Information

Calories 443

Net Carbs 3g

Fats 36.2g

Protein 25.7 g

Fiber 1.7g

Orange Choco-Cashew Smoothie

Serves 1

Ingredients

1 cup cashew milk

1 handful of arugula leaves

1 Tbsp chocolate whey protein powder

1/8 tsp orange extract

Ice cubes

Directions

1. Place all ingredients in your blender and blend until well united and smooth. Add extra ice and serve.

Amount Per Serving

Calories 44,97

Total Fat 1,05g

Total Carbs 7,1g

Fiber 2,49g

Sugar 4,4g

Protein 3,97g

Kale Sausage Omelet Pie

Serves: 8

Ingredients

10 eggs

1 1/2 cup Mahón cheese (or Cheddar)

3 chicken sausages

3 cups raw chopped Kale leaves

2 1/2 cup mushrooms, chopped

1 Tbsp garlic powder

2 tsp Hot sauce

1/2 tsp black pepper and celery seed

salt and pepper to taste

Directions

1. Preheat oven to 400F.
2. Chop up your sausage and mushroom thin and place them in a cast iron skillet. Cook on a medium-high heat for 2-3 minutes.
3. While the sausages are cooking, chop your spinach up. Add in a skillet the mushrooms and spinach.
4. In a meanwhile, in a bowl mix eggs with black pepper and celery seed, hot sauce, and spices. Scramble them well.
5. Mix your sausages, spinach, and mushrooms so that the spinach can wilt fully. Add salt and pepper to taste.
6. Finally, add the cheese to the top.

7. Pour your eggs over the mixture and mix everything well.
8. Stir the mixture for a few seconds, and then put your cast iron skillet in the oven. Bake for 10-12 minutes, and then broil the top for 3-4 minutes.
9. Let cool for a while, cut into 8 slices and serve hot.

Cooking Time: 25 minutes

Amount Per Serving

Calories 266,11

Total Fat 17,76g

Total Carbohydrates 7,67g

Fiber 0,92g

Sugar 1,58g

Protein 19,37g

Bacon, Scallions & Monterey Omelet

Serves: 2

Ingredients

2 eggs

2 slices cooked bacon

1/4 cup scallions, chopped

1/4 cup Monterey jack cheese

salt and pepper to taste

1 tsp lard

Directions

1. In a frying pan heat lard in on medium-low heat. Add the eggs, scallions and salt and pepper to taste.
2. Cook for 1-2 minutes; add the bacon and sauté 30 - 45 seconds longer. Turn the heat off on the stove.
3. On top of the bacon place a cheese. Then, take two edges of the omelet and fold them onto the cheese. Hold the edges there for a moment as the cheese has to partially melt. Make the same with the other egg and let cook in a warm pan for a while.
4. Serve hot.

Cooking Time: 15 minutes

Amount Per Serving

Calories 321,48

68

Total Fat 28,31g

Total Carbs 1,62g

Fiber 0,33g

Sugar 0,55g

Protein 14,37g

Bacon, Avocado & Smoked Turkey Muffins

Serves: 16

Ingredients

5 eggs

6 slices smoked turkey bacon

1/2 cup almond flour

2 medium Avocados

1/2 cup Cheddar cheese

1 1/2 cup coconut milk

3 spring onions

1 tsp minced garlic

2 tsp dried parsley

1/4 tsp red chili powder

1 1/2 Tbsp lemon juice

1/4 cup flaxseed

1 1/2 Tbsp Metamucil powder

1 tsp baking powder

2 Tbsp butter

salt and pepper to taste

Directions

1. Preheat oven to 350F.

2. In a frying pan over medium-low heat, cook the bacon with the butter until crisp. Add the spring onions, cheese, and baking powder.
3. In a bowl, mix together coconut milk, eggs, Metamucil powder, almond flour, flax, spices and lemon juice. Switch off the heat and let cool. Then, crumble the bacon and add all of the fat to the egg mixture.
4. Clean and chop avocado and fold into the mixture.
5. Measure out batter into a cupcake tray that's been sprayed or greased with nonstick spray and bake for 25-26 minutes.
6. Once ready, let cool and serve hot or cold.

Cooking Time: 40 minutes

Amount Per Serving

Calories 184

Total Fat 16,4g

Total Carbs 5,51g

Fiber 2,7g

Sugar 0,54g

Protein 5,89g

Cream Cheese Pancakes

Serves: 16

Ingredients

2 eggs

1/4 cup cream cheese

1 Tbsp coconut flour

1 tsp ground ginger

1/2 cup liquid Stevia

coconut oil

sugar-free maple syrup

Directions

1. In a deep bowl, beat together all of the ingredients until smooth.
2. Heat up a frying skillet with oil on medium-high. Ladle the batter and pour in hot oil.
3. Cook on one side and then flip. Top with a sugar-free maple syrup and serve.

Cooking Time: 15 minutes

Amount Per Serving

Calories 170,78

Total Fat 13,71g

72

Total Carbohydrates 4,39g

Fiber 0,14g

Sugar 1,27g

Protein 6,9g

Chapter 5

Delicious Ketogenic Diet Lunch Recipes

Salmon Salad in Avocado Cups

Ingredients

1 medium-sized salmon fillet

1 pc. shallot, diced

¼ cup mayo

½ juice of lime

2 tsps. fresh dill, chopped

1 tbsp. ghee

1 large avocado, sliced in half and pitted

salt and pepper to taste

Directions

1. Preheat oven at 400F
2. Place the salmon fillet on a baking sheet and drizzle it with ghee and juice of lime. Season with salt and pepper and place in the oven to cook for 20-25 minutes.
3. When done, allow the salmon to cook for a few minutes and shred using a fork.
4. Place the salmon in a bowl, add the diced shallot, and mix well.
5. Add the dill and mayo to the salmon mixture and combine well. Set aside.
6. Remove the insides of the avocado halves making sure that the skin is still intact to make cups.
7. Mash the avocado meat in a bowl and then add to the salmon mixture. Combine well.
8. Transfer the avocado and tuna salad back to the avocado cups and serve.

Nutritional Info (per serving)

Calories:463

Net Carbs: 6.4g

Fat: 35g

Protein: 27g

Cheesy Hotdog Pockets

Ingredients

2 pcs. beef hot dogs

2 thick sticks of quick-melt cheese (or mozzarella)

4 slices of bacon

1/8 tsp. garlic powder

1/8 tsp. onion powder

salt and pepper to taste

Directions

1. Preheat oven at 400F
2. Cut the hotdogs lengthwise to create slits.
3. Insert the cheese sticks in the hotdog and then wrap the bacon with to the beef hotdog. Secure the bacon using a toothpick.
4. Transfer the hotdogs on a baking sheet lined with foil and flavor with garlic and onion powder.
5. Place in the oven to cook for 40 minutes or until the hotdogs turns golden brown and the cheese is melted,
6. Serve with a veggie salad on the side.

Nutritional Info (per serving)

Calories:378

Net Carbs: 0.3 g

Fat: 35g

Protein: 17g

78

Beef Shred Salad

Ingredients

2 cups beef, shredded

1 yellow pepper, sliced thin lengthwise

1 white onion, sliced lengthwise

6 pcs. butter lettuce

2 tsp. mayo

1/8 tsp. chili flakes

Directions

1. Place the butter lettuces on a serving plate. Spread mayo on the lettuce and top with the shredded beef.
2. Place pepper slices and onions on top and season with chili flakes.
3. Serve as it is or rolled.

Nutritional Info (per serving)

Calories: 338

Net Carbs: 2.4

Fat: 25g

Protein: 24g

Homemade Meatballs

Ingredients

500g ground beef

1 whole egg

½ cup almond flour

2 cloves of garlic, minced

1 tsp. oregano, dried

1 tsp. thyme, dried

1 cup mozzarella cheese, shredded

salt and pepper to taste

½ cup homemade marinara sauce

Directions

1. Preheat oven at 450F.
2. In a large bowl, place the ground beef, egg, almond flour, garlic, oregano, thyme, and season with salt and pepper. Also add the cheese.
3. Using your hands, mix all the ingredients together, making sure that everything is well combined.
4. Create 25 pcs of meat balls and lay them on a baking sheet lined with parchment paper.
5. Cook in the oven to cook for 15 minutes or until golden brown.
6. Serve the meatballs with marinara sauce.

Nutritional Info (per serving)

80

Calories: 117

Net Carbs: 0.9

Fat: 9.3g

Protein: 7g

Spicy Chicken Thighs

Ingredients

2 lb. chicken thighs

¼ cup ghee or olive oil

½ tsp garlic powder

½ tsp. paprika

½ tsp. cumin, ground

¼ tsp. cayenne

¼ tsp. coriander, ground

1/8 tsp. cinnamon, ground

1/8 tsp. ginger powder

1 tsp. salt

1 tsp. yellow curry

Directions

1. Preheat oven at 425F.
2. In a small bowl mix all the spices to create a dry rub.
3. Pat dry the chicken using a kitchen paper towel and place on a baking sheet lined with greased parchment paper.
4. Generously brush the chicken with ghee or olive oil.
5. Rub the spices to the chicken thighs making sure that you cover every side.
6. Place the chicken in the oven to cook for 50 minutes.
7. Let it cool before serving.

Nutritional Info (per serving)

Calories:227

Net Carbs: .6g

Fat: 20g

Protein: 21g

Spring Roll in a Bowl

Ingredients

500g pork mince

2 cups cabbage, shredded finely

2 cup grated carrot

2 cups grated baby marrows

1 cup mushrooms

4 tbsp. coconut oil

1/2 cup soya sauce

1 cup chicken stock

2 tsp vinegar

5 cloves garlic, minced

4 tsp grated ginger

4 finely sliced spring onions

½ cup toasted sesame seeds

1 hard-boiled egg, chopped

Directions

1. Heat the coconut oil and fry the garlic, spring onions, ginger.
2. Add the pork mince and brown.
3. Add the cabbage and carrot to the pot and toss to combine. Stir in the soy sauce.
4. Cover and cook until the vegetables are soft, about 15 minutes.

5. Dish up, add chopped hard-boiled egg over each of the bowls.
6. Garnish with sesame seeds once you have dished up.

Nutritional Info (per serving)

Calories: 80

Net Carbs: 5g

Fat: 5g

Protein: 3g

Green Salad

(This salad is the salad that is referred to across other meals)

Ingredients

1 cup green beans, steamed lightly

1 cup broccoli florets, steamed lightly

1 small tomato, finely sliced

1 cup lettuce

1 round feta

¼ cup toasted sunflower seeds, roasted

1 hard-boiled egg, chopped

For dressing:

1 tbsp. olive oil

Salt and pepper to taste

juice from ½ lemon

Directions

1. Place all the vegetables in a salad bowl.
2. Crumble the feta and sprinkle it along with the roasted pumpkin seeds and egg on top of the salad.

3. In a small bowl, pour the olive oil, add lemon juice, then add salt and pepper, and whisk together. Drizzle this dressing on top of the salad.
4. Toss gently before serving.

Nutritional Info (per serving)

Calories:45

Net Carbs: 3g

Fat: 3g

Protein: 1g

Greek Salad

Ingredients

50g Grilled Chicken Breast

2 cups lettuce

10 Olives

½ Round Feta

5 Cherry Tomatoes

¼ Cucumber

1Tblsp Olive Oil

1tsp Lemon juice

Directions

1. Place all ingredients into a bowl, mix and enjoy!

Bacon, Lettuce, Tomato Salad

Ingredients

1 cup of lettuce

1 spring onion

1 tomato

¼ cup toasted pumpkin seeds

grated boiled egg

sliced avocado

4 rashes of crispy bacon(crumbled)

For dressing:

1 Tblsp apple cider vinegar

1 tsp lemon juice

½ a finely crushed clove of garlic

1 Tblsp Olive oil and some finely crushed fresh ginger (optional)

Directions

1. In a large bowl combine salad ingredients
2. This can all be done at home and taken to work.

For dressing:

1. In a separate container mix dressing ingredients
2. Allow the dressing to sit for a few hours.

Pour the dressing over the salad when you are ready to eat.

Broccoli Salad

Ingredients

1 cup broccoli

2 medium celery stalks

1/2 cup mushroom pieces (fried)

1/4 cup Cherry tomatoes

1Tblsp olive oil

2 cups Lettuce

1Tblsp Balsamic Vinegar

125ml pumpkin seeds roasted dry in a pan.

Directions

1. Place all ingredients into a bowl, mix and enjoy!

Tuna/Smoked Salmon Salad

Ingredients

1 Tin Tuna in Water/100g Smoked Salmon

1 Hard Boiled Egg

½ Avo

1 Cup Green Beans (Steamed)

5 Cherry Tomatoes

1 Tblsp Red Onion

½ Cup Celery

Directions

1. Place all ingredients into a bowl, mix and enjoy!

Avo & Tuna Lettuce Wraps

In a medium bowl, combine all ingredients for tuna salad. Mix with a fork. Refrigerate. To assemble, spoon tuna mixture into lettuce leaves. Top with avocado and tomato.

Warm Chicken Salad

Ingredients

1. Roast 2 medium chicken thighs in the oven the night before and remove meat from bones (eat skin whilst warm).

2. Reheat Chicken the following day and add to salad

Hearty Salad

Ingredients

1 Hard Boiled Egg grated

2 slices of country ham, finely sliced

30g cheddar cheese

1 tomato finely diced

2Tblsp Mayo

1 cup finely sliced crispy lettuce

2 spring onions finely chopped

½ green pepper finely chopped

Directions

1. Combine all the ingredients and then add the mayo and mix.

Crunchy Chicken Waldorf Salad

Ingredients

150ml full cream plain yogurt

1Tblsp Mayonnaise

2 teaspoons lemon juice

1/4 teaspoon salt

50g chopped cooked chicken breast

½ medium green apple, finely diced

1 cup finely sliced celery

1/2 cup chopped walnuts, toasted.

Directions

1. Whisk mayonnaise, yogurt, lemon juice and salt in a large bowl.
2. Add chicken, apple, celery and 1/4 cup walnuts.
3. Stir to coat well.
4. Serve topped with the remaining 1/4 cup walnuts.

Savoury Mince

Serves 10

Ingredients

4Tblsp Coconut oil

1Kg Beef/Chicken/Lamb/Pork/Ostrich mince

2 Onion finely diced

4 cups Vegetables (green/red/yellow/orange peppers, mushroom, tomatoes, celery, baby marrows, spinach) finely diced

4 Carrots finely grated

1 Packet gluten free gravy

½ cup Tomato paste

250ml chicken stock

Directions

1. Heat coconut oil in a pan and fry chopped onion,
2. Add beef mince with and tomato paste and fry.
3. Add chopped vegetables and grated carrot to the cooked mince.
4. Continue to cook on a low heat until the vegetables are well cooked.
5. If your mixture seems to be drying out, keep adding chicken stock to keep at the right consistency.
6. The longer you cook this mixture, the more the flavors will infuse through the mince.
7. Add gluten free gravy.

Spinach Cheese & Bacon Log

Serves 5

Ingredients

Cheddar cheese (2 ½ cups, shredded)

Chipotle seasoning (2 tablespoons)

Bacon (30 slices)

Mrs. Dash seasoning (2 teaspoons)

Spinach (5 cups)

Directions

1. Set oven to 375 F.
2. Place bacon in a weaving pattern on a baking sheet lined with foil and season with spices.
3. Top bacon with cheese leaving a 1 inch space all around the edge. Add spinach and push it down and roll the bacon together into a log.
4. Sprinkle with salt and place into oven for 60 minutes.
5. Cool for 15 minutes and slice.
6. Serve.

Nutritional Information

Calories 432

Net Carbs 3g

Fats 38.2g

Protein 32.8 g

Fiber 3g

Beef Sausage, Bacon & Broccoli Casserole

Ingredients

500 g beef sausage

1/2 head of broccoli

8 slices of bacon

Cream (1/2 cups)

Dijon mustard (1 tablespoon)

100 g grated cheddar cheese

Directions

1. Preheat oven to 350F
2. Slice the sausage and place in a small baking dish.
3. Slice the bacon and add to the sausage.
4. Break the broccoli into florets and arrange between the meat.
5. Mix the cream and mustard in a bowl and pour it all over the casserole, then top with the cheese.
6. Bake in the oven for 35 minutes.

Nutritional Information

Calories: 300

Net Carbs: 3g

Fat: 25g

Protein: 20g

Keto Ham & Grilled Cheese Sandwich

Ingredients

For buns:

Eggs (2)

Salted butter (1 ½ tablespoons)

Coconut flour (1 teaspoon)

Almond flour (3/4 cup)

Coconut oil (2 tablespoons)

Baking powder (1 teaspoon)

Salt (1/4 teaspoon)

Filling:

Deli Ham (4 slices)

Cheddar cheese (2 slices)

Butter (1 tablespoon, salted)

Muenster cheese (2 slices)

Directions

1. Set oven to 350 F.
2. Place almond flour, baking powder in a bowl and mix together.
3. Put coconut oil and butter in a microwavable dish and heat until melted then add to dry mix. Combine until mixture gets doughy.

4. Beat eggs and add to dough mixture then put in coconut flour.
5. Grease cupcake molds and add batter to each about ¾ ways filled. Baked for 18 minutes and take from oven, allow to cool and slice into two horizontally.
6. Use cheese and ham to fill buns, melt butter in a skillet and place sandwiches into pan. Cook for 3 minutes on each side until golden and cheese melts.
7. Serve.

Nutritional Information

Calories 272

Net Carbs 1.8g

Fats 24.2g

Protein 11.3g

Fiber 3.8g

Portobello Burgers

Serves 1

Ingredients

Coconut oil (1/2 tablespoon)

Oregano (1 teaspoon)

Portobello mushroom caps (2)

Garlic (1 clove)

Salt

Black pepper

Dijon mustard (1 tablespoon)

Cheddar cheese (1/4 cup)

Beef/bison (6 oz.)

Directions

1. Heat griddle and combine spices and oil in a bowl.
2. Remove gills from mushrooms and place into marinade until needed.
3. Add beef, cheese, salt, mustard and pepper in another bowl and mix to combine; form into a patty.
4. Place marinated caps onto grill and cook for 8 minutes until thoroughly heated. Place patty onto grill and cook on each side for 5 minutes.
5. Take 'buns' from grill and top with burger and any other toppings you choose.
6. Serve.

Nutritional Information

Calories 735

Net Carbs 4g

Fats 48g

Protein 60g

Fiber 4g

Zucchini Stuffed with Chicken & Broccoli

Serves 2

Ingredients

Butter (2 tablespoons)

Broccoli (1 cup)

Sour cream (2 tablespoons)

Zucchini (10 oz.)-2

Cheddar cheese (3 oz., shredded)

Rotisserie chicken (6 oz., shredded)

Green onion (1 stalk)

Salt

Black pepper

Directions

1. Set oven to 400 F.
2. Slice zucchinis in half lengthwise and use spoons to remove cores. Melt butter and pour equally into each zucchini shell. Add black pepper and salt and bake for 20 minutes.
3. Chop broccoli and place into a bowl with sour cream and chicken. Fill zucchini boats with chicken mixture and top with cheese.
4. Bake for 15 minutes more or until golden.
5. Serve topped with green onion.

Nutritional Information

Calories 476.5

Net Carbs 5g

Fats 34g

Protein 30 g

Fiber 3g

Beef Pumpkin Chili

Serves 8

Ingredients

2 lbs ground beef

1 can (15 oz) pumpkin puree

1 Tbs pumpkin pie spice

3 cups 100% tomato juice

3 tomatoes, diced

1 red bell pepper

1 yellow onion

2 tsp cumin

1 Tbs chili powder

2 tsp cayenne pepper

ghee or coconut oil

Directions

1. In a large frying pan greased with ghee or coconut oil, brown the meat over medium heat.
2. Chop the onion and pepper and add into the pot with the meat. Cook 3-5 minutes or until the onions become translucent.
3. Add in the rest of the ingredients and let simmer on LOW for 30 minutes.
4. Season chili with salt and pepper to taste and cook for another 30 minutes.

5. Serve hot.

Cooking Time: 1 hour and 20 minutes

Amount Per Serving

Total Carbs 9,87g

Calories 354,83

Total Fat 25,24g

Fiber 2,14g

Sugar 5,5g

Protein 21,87g

Slow Cooker Chicken Stew

Serves 10

Ingredients

3 lb pot roast

1 lb chicken breast (boiled and shredded)

6 oz Italian sweet sausage

2 cups beef broth

1 cup chicken stock

1/2 medium onion (chopped)

1 can (11 oz) low carb diced tomatoes

1/4 tsp thyme

1/4 tsp celery salt

1 Tbs coconut oil

1 tsp basil

2 tsp dried dill weed

2 tsp garlic powder

2 tsp pepper

1 Tbsp garlic salt

1 tsp minced garlic

1 Tbsp oregano

1 Tbsp powdered buttermilk

4 tsp onion powder

110

4 tsp dried parsley

5 tsp red pepper flakes

2 tsp hot sauce

Directions

1. At the bottom of your Slow Cooker place roast, chicken breast and Italian sausages. Add on the top all other ingredients and stir lightly.
2. Close the lid and cook on LOW for about 6-8 hours.
3. Once ready, flavor to taste with some additional hot sauce, salt and pepper to your own liking and serve hot.

Amount Per Serving

Total Carbs 3,76g 1%

Calories 467,06

Total Fat 36,21g 56%

Fiber 1,03g 4%

Sugar 0,59g

Protein 30,11g 60%

Pecorino Romano Breaded Cutlets

Serves 3

Ingredients

6 pork cutlets

1/2 cup grated Pecorino Romano cheese

2 Tbsp fresh lemon juice

2 Tbsp water

1 Tbsp olive oil

1 Tbsp green pepper, minced

1 Tbsp garlic, minced

salt and ground black pepper to taste

Directions

1. Heat a greasing frying pan to medium.
2. In a bowl pour water, lemon juice, olive oil, minced pepper and garlic. Season the salt and pepper to taste. Mix well.
3. In a separate bowl pour grated Pecorino Romano cheese.
4. Dip each cutlet first in liquid dressing and then in cheese.
5. Cook cutlets in pan for about 15-20 minutes. Serve hot.

Cooking Time: 30 minutes

Amount Per Serving

Total Carbs 2,5g

Calories 395,93

Total Fat 38,78g

Fiber 0,16g

Sugar 0,37g

Protein 9,1g

Garlic Chicken Thighs

Serves 4

Ingredients

4 chicken thighs

16 whole cloves of garlic

2 Tbsp ghee

2 Tbsp juice of one fresh lemon

1 cup of baby carrots

1 onion, cut into quarters

2 tomatoes, cut in half

3 Tbsp garlic olive oil (or extra-virgin olive oil)

oregano

Salt and pepper

Directions

1. Preheat oven to 500F degrees.
2. Grease the bottom of a non-stick frying pan with garlic olive oil (or olive oil). Add in the chicken thighs together.
3. In between the thighs, wedge in the garlic gloves, onions, tomatoes and baby carrots.
4. Pour the lemon juice over the chicken thighs. Drizzle the ghee and garlic oil over the thighs.
5. Sprinkle oregano over the dish and season with salt and pepper to taste.
6. Bake in preheated oven for 25-30 minutes.

7. Reduce heat to 350 and cook for 20 minutes more.
8. Once ready, let cool for 5 minutes on a wire rack and serve hot.

Cooking Time: 1 hour and 5 minutes

Amount Per Serving

Total Carbs 8,97g

Calories 237,52

Total Fat 14,52g

Fiber 1,31g

Sugar 2,67g

Protein 17,68g

Chicken & Cauliflower Lasagna

Serves 10

Ingredients

12 chicken thighs

30 oz chopped cauliflower

6 green onions

1 onion, chopped

1 green pepper

6 bacon Slices

1 cup Cream Cheese

1/2 cup heavy cream

8 oz Pepper Jack Cheese, shredded

8 oz Cheddar Cheese, shredded

1 Tbsp garlic, minced

salt and pepper to taste

Directions

1. Preheat oven to350F.
2. Chop up a head of cauliflower into florets. Cook the cauliflower in the microwave on the vegetable setting. Set aside.
3. In a pan on stovetop, toss the chicken thighs with salt and pepper to taste. Add some water to about mid thigh and cook for 60 minutes. Chop up the onions and peppers and pan fry it.

4. Add all of the other ingredients, reserving 2 oz Cheddar and 2 oz of Pepper Jack Cheese.
5. Add the mixture into a large, greased casserole dish and top with the remaining cheese.
6. Cover with foil and cook for 30 minutes. Serve hot.

Preparation Time: 20 minutes

Cooking Time: 1 hour and 30 minutes

Amount Per Serving

Total Carbs 13,73g

Calories 486,47

Total Fat 35,69g

Fiber 2,2g

Sugar 2,93g

Protein 28,09g

Chapter 6

Irresistible Ketogenic Diet Dinner Recipes

Italian Fish Stew

Ingredients

4 200g Kingklip fish fillets

2 onions, finely chopped

4 garlic cloves, minced

2 tins peeled, chopped tomato

4 tbsp. tomato paste

250ml white wine

½ tsp. parsley, chopped

¼ tsp. dried oregano

salt and pepper to taste

½ cup olive oil

1 cup water

Directions

1. Preheat oven to 360C
2. Sauté onion and garlic on a pot then add tinned tomatoes and tomato paste and stir.
3. Pour the wine, parsley, oregano, salt, pepper, and water. Stir well and bring to a simmer.
4. Let it simmer for 10-15 minutes to reduce and thicken.
5. Meanwhile, place your fish in baking dish.
6. When sauce is nice and thick, pour it over fish and sprinkle with a little extra oregano.

7. Cover the dish with foil and place in the oven to cook for 20 minutes.
8. Take foil off and return to oven uncovered and cook for another 10 minutes.

Tip: If the sauce is a little runny when fish comes out, place sauce in another pot and put on heat to reduce a little more. Then pour back over fish.

Nutritional Info (per serving)

Calories:315

Net Carbs: 12

Fat: 8g

Protein: 37g

Chicken Stir-Fry

Ingredients

4 chicken breasts (butterfly), marinate in egg white overnight

2 cups red pepper

2 cups mange tout

2 cups grated carrot

2 cups broccoli

2 cups almonds

2 cloves of garlic

½ tsp. ginger

2 tbsp. soya sauce

125ml chicken stock.

2 tbsp. coconut oil

Directions

1. Heat coconut oil in a pan over medium fire. Sauté the garlic and ginger until fragrant.
2. Cook the chicken breast in the oil and then add the vegetables. Toss and cook until almost done.
3. Add 2 tbsp. soya sauce and 125ml chicken stock. Allow to simmer uncovered until the broth evaporates.

Nutritional Info (per serving)

Calories:186

Net Carbs: 4g

Fat: 11g

Protein: 17g

Pan Fried Hake

Ingredients

1 tbsp. olive oil

Salt and pepper to taste

1 250g Hake fillet

fresh lemon wedges

Directions

1. Heat the olive oil in a large frying pan over medium-high heat.
2. Pat the fish dry with kitchen paper towel and then season with salt and pepper on both sides.
3. Fry the fish for about 4-5 minutes on each side, depending on their thickness, or until they have a golden crust and the flesh flakes away easily with a fork.

Nutritional Info (per serving)

Calories:170

Net Carbs: 7g

Fat: 8g

Protein: 18g

Creamed Spinach

Ingredients

2 cups spinach

½ small onion, chopped

¼ cup water

½ stock cube

1 clove of garlic, chopped

½ cup heavy cream

2 tbsp. butter

salt and pepper to taste

Directions

1. Place spinach and onion to a pan with water and heat over medium-high fire.
2. Add stock cube and garlic and allow to steam for 8-10 minutes or until all the water has evaporated and the spinach is very soft.
3. Pour in the heavy cream and butter and then season with salt and pepper. Cooking until it thickens.
4. Using a hand-held blender blitz the spinach until fairly smooth.
5. Serve while hot

Nutritional Info (1/2 cup)

Calories: 200

Net Carbs: 3g

Fat: 23g

Protein: 7g

Chicken and Mushroom Stew

Ingredients

8 pcs. chicken thighs

4 tbsp. butter

3 cloves garlic, minced

6 cups mushrooms

1 cup chicken stock

½ tsp. dried thyme

½ tsp. dried oregano

½ tsp. dried basil

¼ cup heavy cream

½ cup parmesan cheese, grated

1 tbsp. whole-grain mustard

Directions

1. Preheat oven to 400F
2. Season chicken thighs with salt and pepper
3. Heat an oven-proof pan over medium fire and melt 2 tbsp. of butter.
4. Add the chicken, skin-side down, and fry both sides until golden brown, or about 2-3 minutes per side. Set aside.
5. Melt remaining 2 tbsp. butter. Add garlic, thyme, oregano and basil and mushrooms, and cook, stirring occasionally. Cook until browned, about 5-6 minutes, season with salt and pepper, to taste.
6. Stir in chicken stock, then chicken back to the pan.

7. Pour everything into a baking dish with the chicken.
8. Place into oven and roast until completely cooked through for about 25-30 minutes. Set aside chicken.
9. Transfer sauces back into the original pan.
10. Stir in heavy cream, parmesan cheese and mustard. Bring to a boil; reduce heat and simmer until slightly reduced, about 5 minutes.
11. Serve chicken immediately, topped with mushroom mixture.

Nutritional Info (1 serving)

Calories: 203

Net Carbs: 9g

Fat: 3g

Protein: 28g

Beef Shin Stew

Ingredients

2 lb. quality shin of beef

4 tbsp. olive oil

2 red onions, peeled and roughly chopped

3 pcs. carrots, peeled and roughly chopped

3 sticks celery, trimmed and roughly chopped

4 cloves garlic, unpeeled

a few sprigs of fresh rosemary

2 bay leaves

2 cups mushrooms

2 cups baby marrows

salt and pepper to taste

1 tbsp. psyllium husk

2 cans 400 g tomatoes

⅔ bottle red wine

Directions

1. Preheat your oven to 360F
2. In a heavy-bottomed oven-proof saucepan, heat olive oil and sauté the onions, carrots, celery, garlic, herbs, and mushrooms for 5 minutes until softened slightly.
3. Meanwhile, toss the pieces of beef in the psyllium husk, shaking off any excess.

4. Add the meat to the pan and stir everything together.
5. Add the tomatoes, wine and a pinch of salt and pepper and gently bring to the boil.
6. Turn off heat then cover the sauce pan with a double-thickness piece of tinfoil and a lid and place in oven to cook for 3 hours or until the beef is meltingly tender and can be broken up with a spoon.
7. Taste and check the seasoning, remove the rosemary sprigs and serve hot.

Nutritional Info (1 serving)

Calories: 315

Net Carbs: 7g

Fat: 7g

Protein: 20g

Bacon, Beef Sausage and Broccoli Casserole

Ingredients

500 g beef sausage

1/2 head of broccoli

8 slices of bacon

1/2 cup of cream

1 tbsp. Dijon mustard

100 g grated cheddar cheese

Directions

1. Preheat oven to 350F
2. Slice the sausage and place in a small baking dish.
3. Slice the bacon and add to the sausage.
4. Break the broccoli into florets and arrange between the meat.
5. Mix the cream and mustard in a bowl and pour it all over the casserole, then top with the cheese.
6. Bake in the oven for 35 minutes.

Nutritional Info (1 serving)

Calories: 300

Net Carbs: 3g

Fat: 25g

Protein: 20g

Creamy Haddock

Ingredients

150g smoked haddock

100ml boiling water

1 tbsp. butter

50ml cream

2 cups spinach

Directions

1. Heat a saucepan over medium fire.
2. Mix the boiling water with cream and butter in a bowl.
3. Place haddock and sauce in the pan and leave to boil until the water evaporates, leaving a creamy, butter sauce behind.
4. Serve haddock, covered with the sauce on fresh or wilted spinach.

Nutritional Info (1 serving)

Calories: 281

Net Carbs: 15g

Fat: 10g

Protein: 18g

Cauliflower Bake

Ingredients

4 slices of bacon

2 cups broccoli

2 cups cauliflower

2 cups mushrooms

1 green pepper

1 onion

200ml cream

120g cheese, grated

2 tbsp. olive oil

Directions

1. Preheat oven at 360F.
2. Steam or cook the cauliflower and broccoli until tender then transfer in an oven-proof dish.
3. Fry the bacon slices, with the mushrooms, green pepper and onion in 2 tbsp. olive oil.
4. Pour the fried bacon and mushrooms on top of cauliflower.
5. In a bowl, whisk 4 eggs with the cream and season to taste and pour over cauliflower or broccoli.
6. Place in the oven to cook for 25 minutes. Take out of the oven and sprinkle with grated cheese.
7. Place back in the oven and cook for another 5 minutes.

Nutritional Info (1 serving)

Calories: 100

Net Carbs: 7g

Fat: 6g

Protein: 4g

Caulicake

Ingredients

600 g cauliflower florets

1 onion, chopped

3 cloves of garlic, finely chopped

1 tsp turmeric

100g parmesan cheese, finely grated

100g mature white cheddar cheese, coarsely grated

8 eggs

1-2 tsp. salt

2 tbsp. psyllium husk

1 cup of cream

1 tbsp. coconut oil

sesame seeds

olive oil

Directions

1. Preheat oven at 360F
2. Steam the cauliflower. Keep half of it whole and mash the rest.
3. Sauté the onion, garlic, turmeric in the coconut oil until soft. Set aside.

4. In a separate bowl, whisk the eggs. Add the cream, cheese, salt, and psyllium husk.
5. Combine the cauliflower, whole and mashed with the sautéed onions and egg mixture in a bowl.
6. Line a spring-form baking tin with greased baking paper and sprinkle with sesame seeds. Place the pan onto a baking tray.
7. Pour in the cauliflower mix and bake in the oven for 40 minutes.
8. As soon as it comes out of the oven, lightly prick the surface all over with a fork and drizzle with olive oil.

Nutritional Info (1 serving)

Calories: 160

Net Carbs: 5g

Fat: 11g

Protein: 8g

Keto Burger Patties

Ingredients

500g ground beef

1 small onion, finely chopped

1 red pepper, chopped

¼ cup cheese, grated

1 carrot, grated

1 baby marrow, grated

1 tsp. ginger, grated

1 tsp. crushed garlic

2 eggs

2 tbsp. almond flour

1 tsp. parsley, minced

1 tsp. coriander

Salt and pepper to take

Directions

1. Mix all ingredients together in a bowl.
2. Form the mixture into balls and flatten into patties.
3. Roll the patties in almond flour and leave to firm in the fridge for around 30 mins. This will help to keep the patties from falling apart while cooking.
4. When firm, pan fry the patties in coconut oil. Make sure your oil is hot before adding patties to the pan, you need to hear that oil sizzle. If the oil

is not hot, the patty will stick to the pan and fall apart while cooking.

5. Take 1 large brown mushroom, rub with olive oil and some crushed garlic, do not salt. And bake in the oven at 360F for 15-20mins. Place the cooked burger on top of the mushroom, add grated cheese and melt in the oven for a couple of minutes.

6. Add 1 tbsp. mayo to finely diced red onion, lettuce and tomato and place on top of burger.

Nutritional Info (1 serving)

Calories: 340

Net Carbs: 3g

Fat: 28g

Protein: 17g

Easy, Peasy, Cheese Pizza

Ingredients

2 whole eggs

1 cup cheddar cheese, grated

1 tbsp. psyllium husk

3 tbsp. pesto sauce

Directions

1. Preheat oven at 350F.
2. Mix eggs and cheese along with the psyllium husk in a bowl and combine well.
3. Place the mixture on baking paper and spread quite thinly. Place in the oven to cook for 15-20 minutes. Remember to keep an eye on it, as it gets brown and crispy quickly relative to the thickness, don't make it too thin.
4. Once cooked, remove from the oven and place whatever you wish over the base, like the pesto sauce or tomato sauce.
5. Top with your favorite pizza toppings such as bacon slices, pepperoni chicken, fresh tomato, and fresh basil.

Nutritional Info (1 serving)

Calories: 335

Net Carbs: 3.2g

Fat: 27g

Protein: 18g

Slow Cooker Oxtail Stew

Serves 10

Ingredients

1.5kg of oxtail

1 Large pack grated cabbage

1 Large pack grated carrots

2 Large onions

1 Large Bunch of celery

1 Tin of tomatoes

2 Jelly Stock Cubes

2.5 litres of water

1Tblsp Crushed garlic

1 branch Rosemary

2 Bay Leaves

Directions

1. Place all ingredients into a slow cooker and cook on medium for 9 hours. Season with salt and pepper
2. Grate 60g cheddar cheese to finish (optional).

Chicken Hash

Ingredients

1 Tblsp olive oil

1/4 onion finely diced

1 cups broccoli

1 cup chicken stock

50g chicken breast cooked and finely diced

½ tsp salt

¼ tsp black pepper

¼ cup pumpkin

Directions

1. Add all ingredients to chicken stock, cover and cook approximately 20 minutes

Tuna Fish Stew

Ingredients

1 tin tuna in water, drained

1 Tblsp butter

¼ small onion, chopped finely

1 clove garlic, minced

1teaspoon fresh ginger, grated

½ tin tomatoes, chopped finely

1 cup spinach, chopped finely

1 small carrot, grated

1 teaspoon curry powder 1 teaspoon turmeric

½ teaspoon cayenne pepper (optional)

Salt & pepper to taste

Directions

1. Fry onion, garlic and ginger in butter.
2. Add tomatoes once onions are soft.
3. Add spices and enough water to make a stew for the spinach, carrot and tuna fish. Cook at low heat for about 15 minutes.
4. Do not overcook spinach.
5. Steam 2 cups of cauliflower, mash and add 1Tblsp of butter. Serve stew on top of the caulimash.

Ratatouille

Serves 4

Ingredients

2 large brinjals

1 large onion

2 peppers (can be green, red, yellow)

2 tins of chopped tomatoes

1 packet baby marrows

1 punnet mushrooms

1 packet spinach

500ml chicken stock

Salt & pepper

2 cloves garlic (finely chopped or pressed)

Directions

1. Finely chop all the ingredients.
2. Add all the finely chopped veggies, garlic and onion to the stock and boil on medium until the water has reduced, and the veggies have formed a thick delicious stew.
3. Serve with 150g chunky cottage cheese, 30g cheddar or 6Tblsp Parmesan Cheese

145

Easy Roast Tomato Sauce

Serves 10

Ingredients

10 tomatoes

Bunch of fresh bazil

Garlic, bulb

Olive oil

Salt and pepper

Directions

1. Preheat oven to 190C,
2. Slice 10 tomatoes in half lengthways
3. Add a bunch of fresh basil.
4. Cut an entire bulb of garlic through the middle and place each half face up in the baking tray/dish
5. Immerse the tomatoes in olive oil and grind salt and pepper (Himalayan).
6. Roast in oven for about 1 hour and then turn the oven off for another 30 mins and leave to sit in the warm oven.
7. Remove the tomatoes and allow to cool,
8. do not mix, as you want to squeeze the flesh and pips out of the skin and discard the skin, squeeze the garlic from the cloves and throw away the casings.
9. Mash with a fork

Note: This makes THE best roast tomato sauce for pizza's meatballs or any other protein. Freeze in small Ziploc bags or plastic containers.

You can add onion, red and yellow peppers and fresh chill for more robust flavour. Use a hand blender to blitz if you want a smoother sauce.

Tender Pork & Bacon Cassoulet

Serves 4

Ingredients

1 pack bacon, fried and then crumbled

Chopped onion (2 cups)

Dried thyme (1 teaspoon)

Dried rosemary (1/2 teaspoon)

3 garlic cloves, crushed

Salt (1/2 teaspoon)

Freshly ground black pepper (1/2 teaspoon)

2 cans diced tomatoes, drained

500g boneless pork loin roast, trimmed and cut into 2cm cubes

250g smoked sausage, cut into 1cm cubes

Finely shredded fresh Parmesan cheese (8 teaspoons)

Chopped fresh flat-leaf parsley (8 teaspoons)

Directions

1. Fry bacon onion, thyme, rosemary, and garlic, then add salt, pepper, and tomatoes; bring to a boil.
2. Remove from heat.
3. Place all ingredients in the slow cooker, alternating the meat with the tomato sauce until finished. Cover and cook on low for 5 hours.

148

Sprinkle with Parmesan cheese and parsley when cooked

Nutritional Information

Calories- 258

Carbs- 10.8g

Protein- 27g

Fats- 12.6g

Orange Glazed Duck

Serves 1

Ingredients

Butter (2 tablespoons)

Swerve (1 tablespoon)

Sage (1/4 teaspoon)

Duck breast (6 oz.)

Heavy cream (1 tablespoon)

Orange extract (1/2 teaspoon)

Spinach (1 cup)

Directions

1. Use knife to score the skin of the duck and season with black pepper and salt.
2. Add Swerve and butter to a pot and cook until slightly golden then add extract and sage. Cook until butter has darkened.
3. In another pot, place chicken breast with skin side down and place over a medium flame and cook until skin is crisp.
4. Flip over and add cream to sage mixture and pour over duck. Cook until duck is done.
5. Add spinach to pot and cook until wilted.
6. Serve.

Nutritional Information

Calories 798

Net Carbs 0g

Fats 71g

Protein 36 g

Fiber 1g

Chicken, Bacon & Cream Cheese Pot Pie

Serves 8

Ingredients

For filling:

Bacon (5 slices)

Garlic powder (1 teaspoon)

Cream cheese (8 oz.)

Spinach (6 cups)

Salt

Chicken thighs (6, boneless and skinless)

Onion powder (1 teaspoon)

Celery seed (3/4 teaspoon)

Cheddar cheese (4 oz.)

Chicken broth (1/4 cup)

For crust:

Psyllium Husk Powder (3 tablespoons)

Eggs (1)

Cheddar cheese (1/4 cup)

Garlic powder (1/4 teaspoon)

Salt

Almond flour (1/3 cup)

Butter (3 tablespoons)

152

Cream cheese (1/4 cup)

Paprika (1/2 teaspoon)

Onion powder (1/4 teaspoon)

Black pepper

Directions

1. Cube chicken and season with black pepper and salt.
2. Set oven to 375 F.
3. Use spices to season chicken and place into an oven proof skillet and place onto fire and cook until golden on the outside. Add bacon to pan and cook until golden.
4. Add broth to pan along with cheeses and stir to combine. Put in spinach in pan and cook until wilted.
5. Combine dry ingredients for crust in a bowl and add cheddar and cream cheese to a microwave safe dish and then add cheese and combine. Add mixture to dry ingredients and mix together.
6. Form crust, stir ingredients in pot and top with crust and use fork to pierce crust all over.
7. Bake for 15 minutes, take from oven and cool.
8. Serve.

Nutritional Information

Calories 434

Net Carbs 3.4g

Fats 35.6g

Protein 20.4 g

Fiber 3.6g

Chicken Parmesan

Serves 4

Ingredients

For Chicken:

Chicken breasts (3)

Mozzarella cheese (1 cup)

Salt

Black pepper

For coating:

Flaxseed meal (1/4 cup)

Oregano (1 teaspoon)

Black pepper (1/2 teaspoon)

Garlic powder (1/2 teaspoon)

Egg (1)

Pork rinds (2.5 oz.)

Parmesan cheese (1/2 cup)

Salt (1/2 teaspoon)

Red pepper flakes (1/4 teaspoon)

Paprika (2 teaspoons)

Chicken broth (1 ½ teaspoons)

For Sauce:

Tomato sauce (1 cup, low carb)

Garlic (2 cloves)

Salt

Olive oil (1/2 cup)

Oregano (1/2 teaspoon)

Black pepper

Directions

1. Add flax meal, spices, pork rinds and parmesan cheese in a processor and grind until combined.
2. Pound chicken breast and whisk egg with broth in a container. Add all ingredients for sauce to a pan, stir and put over a low flame to cook.
3. Dip chicken in egg and then coat with dry mixture.
4. Heat oil in a pan and fry chicken then transfer to a casserole dish. Top with sauce and mozzarella and bake for 10 minutes.
5. Serve.

Nutritional Information

Calories 646

Net Carbs 4g

Fats 46.8g

Protein 49.3g

Fiber 2.8g

Bell Peppers Stuffed

Serves 4

Ingredients

Ground beef (1 lb.)

Spring onions (2, sliced)

Ginger (2 teaspoons, diced)

Eggs (8)

Bell peppers (2, cut in half)

Garlic (2 teaspoons, diced)

Salt

Black pepper

For Sauce:

Rice wine vinegar (1 ½ tablespoons)

Chili paste (1 tablespoon)

Apricot preserves (1/3 cup, sugar free)

Ketchup (1 tablespoon, low sugar)

Soy sauce (1 tablespoon)

Directions

1. Season beef with pepper and salt and start cooking over a medium flame until browned. Add ginger and garlic and stir together.
2. Push beef to one side and put in spring onions, cook for 2 minutes then stir together with beef. Take from flame and put aside.
3. Add all sauce ingredients to a pan and cook for 3 minutes then add half to beef.
4. Stir sauce and beef together and use to stuff peppers.
5. Set oven to 350 F and bake for 15 minutes.
6. Top with reserved sauce and serve.

Nutritional Information

Calories 470

Net Carbs 6.3g

Fats 35g

Protein 32.3g

Fiber 5.3g

Spicy Mexican Meatballs

Serves 6

Ingredients

1 lb ground beef (92% lean)

4 oz white onion, minced

4 oz Monterey Jack cheese with spicy peppers

1 Tbsp butter

3 cloves garlic

1 1 tsp chili powder

1 1 tsp ground cumin

1 tsp ground coriander

1 egg

sea salt and freshly ground pepper to taste

Directions

1. Preheat oven to 350 degrees.
2. In a frying pan, sauté onions in butter until translucent. Set aside
3. Shred and mince the Monterey Jack cheese with spicy peppers. Set aside.
4. In a mixing bowl, whisk egg with ricotta cheese. Add the spices, salt, and pepper and mix.
5. Add onions and minced Monterey Jack cheese with spicy peppers. Mix well.
6. Add beef and mix until all ingredients are combined.

7. Roll the meat mix into a ball.
8. Place the meatballs on a cookie sheet, and bake about 20 minutes.
9. Serve hot.

Cooking Time: 35 minutes

Amount Per Serving

Total Carbs 2,94g

Calories 321,28

Total Fat 25,25g

Fiber 0,9g

Sugar 0,81g

Protein 19,54g

Lamb Cutlets with Garlic Sauce

Serves 6

Ingredients

4 lbs. lamb cutlets

1 small head of garlic, cloves peeled

2 Tbsp apple cider vinegar

1/2 cup water

1/4 cup extra virgin olive oil

pinch salt and black ground pepper to taste

Directions

1. Crush the garlic cloves thoroughly in a mortar. In a bowl, add the vinegar and water and mix it well with the crushed garlic. Set aside.
2. In a large frying pan, pour the olive oil and fry the lamb cutlets until nicely brown.
3. Add the garlic mixture and let it cook gently for about 10 minutes.
4. Shake the frying pan to spread the garlic mixture evenly over the lamb.
5. Season with salt and black pepper to taste. Serve.

Cooking Times: 40 minutes

Amount Per Serving

Total Carbs 0,16g

Calories 416,68

Total Fat 28,76g

Fiber 0,01g

Sugar 0,05g

Protein 36,68g

Almond Bread

Serves 8

Ingredients

2 eggs

1 cup almond butter, unsalted

3/4 cup almond flour

1 Tbsp cinnamon

1 tsp pure vanilla extract

1/4 tsp baking soda

2 Tbsp liquid Stevia

1/2 tsp sea salt

Directions

1. Preheat oven to 340F degrees.
2. In a deep bowl whisk eggs, almond butter, honey, Stevia and vanilla. Add in salt, cinnamon and baking soda. Stir until all ingredients are well combined.
3. Pour dough in a greased baking pan. Bake for 12-15 minutes.
4. Once ready, let cool on a wire rack. Slice and serve.

Cooking Time: 25 minutes

Amount Per Serving

Total Carbs 7,64g 3%

Calories 208,06

Total Fat 16,7g 26%

Fiber 3,63g 15%

Sugar 1,87g

Protein 7,7g 15%

Tangy Shrimp Soup

Serves 8

Ingredients

12 oz fresh shrimp, peeled and deveined

1 cup zucchini (medium, sliced)

1 onion, chopped

2 cloves garlic, minced

1 Tbsp ginger, minced

1 pinch crushed red pepper

2 quarts water

1 cup celery (chopped)

2 cups cauliflower florets

2 Tbsp soy sauce

1/4 tsp ground black pepper

2 tsp olive oil

Directions

1. In a large saucepan with over medium heat cook onion, garlic, ginger and crushed red pepper for 2 minutes.

2. Pour in water, cauliflower florets and celery and bring to a boil. Reduce heat, cover and simmer 5 minutes.

3. Stir in zucchini and shrimp, season with salt and pepper to taste; cover and cook 5 - 7 minutes.

4. Stir in soy sauce and pepper and serve.

Cooking Times

Total Time: 25 minutes

Amount Per Serving

Total Carbs 7,12g 2%

Calories 107,62

Total Fat 3,08g 5%

Fiber 1,6g 6%

Sugar 3,35g

Protein 12,08g 24%

Baked Herb Salmon Fillets

Serves 6

Ingredients

2 lbs salmon fillets

1/2 cup chopped fresh mushrooms

1/2 cup chopped green onions

4 oz butter

4 Tbsp coconut oil

1/2 cup tamari soy sauce

1 tsp minced garlic

1/4 tsp thyme

1/2 tsp rosemary

1/4 tsp tarragon

1/2 tsp ground ginger

1/2 tsp basil

1 tsp oregano leaves

Directions

1. Preheat oven to 350 degrees F. Line a large baking pan with foil.
2. Cut salmon filet in pieces. Put the salmon into the ziploc bag with the tamari sauce, sesame oil and spices sauce mixture. Refrigerate the salmon and marinade it for 4 hours.

3. Put the salmon in a baking pan and bake fillets for 10-15 minutes.
4. Melt the butter. Add the chopped fresh mushrooms and green onion to it, and mix. Remove the salmon from the oven, and pour the butter mixture over the salmon fillets, making sure each fillet gets covered.
5. Bake for about 10 minutes more. Serve immediately.

Cooking Times

Inactive Time: 4 hours

Total Time: 35 minutes

Amount Per Serving

Total Carbs 2,77g

Calories 449,77

Total Fat 34,11g

Fiber 0,72g

Sugar 0,79g

Protein 33,19g

Kale & Chili "Meatballs"

Serves 8

Ingredients

4 Tbsp olive oil

1 cup almond flour

1 bunch of kale leaves

1 green chili, chopped

1/4 tsp red chili powder

1/4 tsp turmeric powder

1 tsp cumin seed powder

1/4 tsp ginger, minced

black salt or salt as per taste

1 tsp cooking soda or baking soda (optional)

water for batter

Directions

1. In a bowl, mix all the ingredients together.
2. Combine and knead the batter with your finger. The consistency should be nor too thick nor too thin. Make a kale "meatballs".
3. Heat oil in a frying pan. Place a kale "meatballs" in the hot oil one by one.
4. Fry few at a time don't cluster with too many. When they get golden color from one side, turn and cook from another side.

168

5. Remove the fries with slotted spoon and place over absorbent napkins.
6. Serve hot.

Cooking Time: 25 minutes

Amount Per Serving

Total Carbs 13,01g 4%

Calories 125,94

Total Fat 6,24g 10%

Fiber 4,85g 19%

Sugar 0,8g

Protein 6,04g 12%

Chapter 7

Scrumptious Ketogenic Diet Dessert & Snack Recipe

Pecan Blondies

Serves 16

Ingredients

3 eggs

2 1/4 cups pecans, roasted

3 Tbs heavy cream

1 Tbs salted caramel syrup

1/2 cup flax seeds, ground

1/4 cup butter, melted

1/4 cup erythritol, powdered

10 drops Liquid Stevia

1 tsp baking powder

1 pinch salt

Directions

1. Preheat oven to 350F.
2. In a baking pan roast pecans for 10 minutes.
3. Grind 1/2 cup flax seeds in a spice grinder. Place flax seed powder in a bowl. Grind Erythritol in a spice grinder until powdered. Set in the same bowl as the flax seeds meal.
4. Place 2/3 of roasted pecans in food processor and process until a smooth nut butter is formed.
5. Add eggs, liquid Stevia, salted caramel syrup, and a pinch of salt to the flax seed mixture. Mix well. Add pecan butter to the batter and mix again.

172

6. Smash the rest of the roasted pecans into chunks. Add crushed pecans and 1/4 cup melted butter into the batter.
7. Mix batter well, and then add heavy cream and baking powder. Mix everything together well.
8. Place the batter into baking tray and bake for 20 minute. Let cool for about 10 minutes. Slice off the edges of the brownie to create a uniform square. Serve.

Cooking Time: 40 minutes

Amount Per Serving

Total Carbs 3,54g

Calories 180,45

Total Fat 18,23g

Fiber 1,78g

Sugar 1,45g

Protein 3,07g

Chocolate Minty Ice Cream

Serves 3

Ingredients

1/2 tsp Peppermint extract

1 cup heavy cream

1 cup cheese cream

1 tsp pure vanilla extract

1 tsp Liquid Stevia extract

100% Dark Chocolate for topping

Directions

1. Place ice cream bowl in freezer per ice cream maker instructions. In a metal bowl, put all ingredients except chocolate and whisk well.
2. Put back in freezer for 5 minutes. Setup ice cream maker and add liquid.
3. Before serving, top the ice cream with chocolate shavings. Serve.

Cooking Time: 35 minutes

Amount Per Serving

Total Carbs 2,7g

Calories 286,66

Total Fat 29,96g

Fiber 0g

Sugar 0,9g

Protein 2,6g

Coconut Waffles

Serves 8

Ingredients

1 cup coconut flour

1/2 cup heavy (whipping) cream

5 eggs

1/4 tsp pink salt

1/4 tsp baking soda

1/4 cup coconut milk

2 tsp Yacon Syrup (or some other natural sweetener)

2 Tbsp coconut oil (melted)

Directions

1. In a large bowl add the eggs and beat with an electric hand mixer for 30 seconds.
2. Add the heavy (whipping) cream and coconut oil into the eggs while you are still mixing. Add the coconut milk, coconut flour, pink salt and baking soda. Mix with the hand mixer for 45 second on low speed. Set aside.
3. Heat up your waffle maker well and make the waffles according to your manufactures specifications.
4. Serve hot.

Amount Per Serving

Calories 169,21

Total Fat 12,6g 19%

Total Carbs 9,97g 3%

Fiber 0,45g 2%

Sugar 0,38g

Protein 4,39g 9%

Choc- Raspberry Cream

Serves 4

Ingredients

1/2 cup 100% dark chocolate, chopped

1/4 cup of heavy cream

1/2 cup cream cheese, softened

2 Tbsp sugar free Raspberry Syrup

1/4 cup Erythritol

Directions

1. In a double boiler melt chopped chocolate and the cream cheese. Add the Erythritol sweetener and continue to stir. Remove from heat, let cool and set aside.
2. When the cream has cooled add in heavy cream and Raspberry syrup and stir well.
3. Pour cream in a bowls or glasses and serve. Keep refrigerated.

Cooking Time: 15 minutes

Amount Per Serving

Total Carbs 7,47g 2%

Calories 157,67

Total Fat 13,51g 21%

178

Fiber 1g 4%

Sugar 5,16g

Protein 1,95g 4%

Hazelnut & Cacao Cookies

Serves 24

Ingredients

2 cups almond flour

1 cup chopped hazelnut

1/2 cup cacao powder

1/2 cup ground flax

3 Tbsp coconut oil (melted)

1/3 cup water

1/3 cup Erythritol

1/4 tsp liquid Stevia

Directions

1. In a bowl, mix almond flour and flax and cacao powder. Stir in oil, water, agave and vanilla. When it is well mixed, stir in chopped hazelnuts.
2. Form in to balls, press flat with palms and place on dehydrator screens.
3. Dehydrate 1 hour at 145, then reduce to 116 and dehydrate for at least 5 hours or until desired dryness is achieved.
4. Serve.

Cooking Time: 6 hours

Amount Per Serving

Total Carbs 8,75g

Calories 181,12

Total Fat 15,69g

Fiber 3,45g

Sugar 3,75g

Protein 4,46g

Dark Chocolate Brownies

Serves 16

Ingredients

3 eggs

4 oz dark chocolate, unsweetened

1/2 cup coconut oil

1 cup almond flour

1 cup walnuts

2 Tbs cocoa, unsweetened

1 tsp vanilla essence

2 cups granulated sweetener Stevia or Erythritol

1 tsp baking soda

pinch of salt

Directions

1. Preheat the oven to 350F.
2. In a container, add almond flour, sweetener, cocoa, salt and baking soda. With an electric mixer, blend the ingredients on the slowest setting until combined well.
3. Melt the chocolate and the coconut oil together (In a microwave or double boiler). Stir thoroughly.
4. Add eggs and vanilla essence to the flour and mix on a medium speed until a thick batter is formed.

5. Add the butter/chocolate mix to the batter continuing on medium speed until an even texture is formed. Line a slice tin or square baking tin with wax paper. Fold in walnut pieces then turn the batter into your slice tin.
6. Bake for 25 minutes. When ready let cool on wire rack.
7. Cut into 16 Brownies and serve.

Cooking Times

Total Time: 35 minutes

Amount Per Serving

Total Carbs 5,38g

Calories 207,88

Total Fat 20,72g

Fiber 2,82g

Sugar 0,73g

Protein 5,14g

Lemon Squares & Coconut Cream

Serves 8

Ingredients

Base:

3/4 cup coconut flakes

2 Tbsp coconut oil

1 Tbsp ground almonds

Cream:

5 eggs

1/2 lemon juice

1 Tbsp coconut flour

1/2 cup Stevia sweetener

Directions

For the base

1. Preheat oven to 360F.
2. In a bowl put all base ingredients and with clean hands mix everything well until soft.
3. With coconut oil grease a rectangle oven dish. Pour dough in a baking pan. Bake for 15 minutes until golden brown. Set aside to cool.

For the cream

1. In a bowl or blender, whisk together: eggs, lemon juice, coconut flour and sweetener. Pour over the baked caked evenly.
2. Put pan in the oven and bake 20 minutes more.
3. When ready refrigerate for at least 6 hours. Cut in cubes and serve.

Cooking Times

Total Time: 1 hour and 5 minutes

Nutrition Facts (per serving)

Total Carbohydrates: 4g

Dietary Fiber: 2,25g

Net Carbs: 1,4g

Protein: 5g

Total Fat: 15g

Calories: 129

Rich Almond Butter Cake & Chocolate Sauce

Serves 12

Ingredients

1 cup almond butter or soaked almonds

1/4 cup almond milk, unsweetened

1 cup coconut oil

2 tsp liquid Stevia sweetener to taste

Topping: Chocolate Sauce

4 Tbsp cocoa powder, unsweetened

2 Tbsp almond butter

2 Tbsp Stevia sweetener

Directions

1. Melt the coconut oil in room temperature.
2. Add all ingredients in a bowl and blend well until combined.
3. Pour the almond butter mixture into a parchment lined platter.
4. Place in refrigerator for 3 hours.
5. In a bowl, whisk all topping ingredients together. Pour over the almond cake after it's been set. Cut into cubes and serve.

Cooking Time: 5 minutes

Nutrition Facts (per serving)

Total Carbohydrates: 9,8g

Dietary Fiber: 2g

Net Carbs:2,4g

Protein: 5,8g

Total Fat: 23,3g

Calories: 273

Peanut Butter Cake Covered in Chocolate Sauce

Serves 12

Ingredients

1 cup peanut butter

1/4 cup almond milk, unsweetened

1 cup coconut oil

2 tsp liquid Stevia sweetener to taste

Topping: Chocolate Sauce

2 Tbsp coconut oil, melted

4 Tbsp cocoa powder, unsweetened

2 Tbsp Stevia sweetener

Directions

1. In a microwave bowl mix coconut oil and peanut butter; melt in a microwave for 1-2 minutes.
2. Add this mixture to your blender; add in the rest of the ingredients and blend well until combined.
3. Pour the peanut mixture into a parchment lined loaf pan or platter.
4. Refrigerate for about 3 hours; the longer, the better.
5. In a bowl, whisk all topping ingredients together. Pour over the peanut candy after it's been set. Cut into cubes and serve.

Cooking Time: 5 minutes

Nutrition Facts (per serving)

Total Carbohydrates: 5,8g

Dietary Fiber: 2g

Net Carbs: 2,4g

Protein: 6g

Total Fat: 27g

Calories: 273

Spicy Pumpkin Ice Cream

Serves 6

Ingredients

1 cup almond milk (unsweetened)

1 cup coconut milk

1 cup pumpkin puree

2 1/2 tsp ground cinnamon

1 tsp pure vanilla extract

1/2 tsp ground ginger

1/2 tsp nutmeg

1/8 tsp sea salt

Thickener:

1/2 tsp guar gum or 1 tablespoon gelatin dissolved in 1/4 cup boiling water

Directions

1. Put the coconut milk in a blender and purée until smooth.
2. Pour into the ice cream machine or blender and churn well. Serve in chilled glasses.
3. Freeze for about an hour or refrigerate until cold.
4. Add the almond milk, pumpkin puree, vanilla, cinnamon, ginger, nutmeg and salt, plus thickener. Purée until smooth.
5. Serve.

Cooking Times

Inactive Time: 1 hour

Total Time: 15 minutes

Amount Per Serving

Total Carbs 4,73g

Calories 118,25

Total Fat 11,3g

Fiber 1,4g 6%

Sugar 1,43g

Protein 1,35g

Bacon & Onion Bites

Serves 12

Serving Size: 1 cookie

Ingredients

Almond flour (1 ½ cups)

Flax meal (1/3 cup)

Psyllium husk powder (1 tablespoon)

Onion powder (1 tablespoon)

1 large egg

4 slices bacon, cooked until crispy and crumbled

Sea salt (1/2 teaspoon)

Freshly ground pepper

Directions

1. Place all of the dry ingredients into a bowl (almond flour, flax meal, psyllium husk powder, onion powder, salt and pepper) and mix until well combined.
2. If you don't have onion powder, you can use dried onion flakes and blend them until powdered. Also, make sure you don't use whole psyllium husks - blend the psyllium husks until powdered if needed.
3. Add the egg and mix well using your hands.
4. Add the crumbled bacon to the dough. Process well using your hands. (Be sure to save the bacon fat from the cooking process for other uses - like some of the other fat bomb recipes in this book.)

5. Using your hand, create 12 equal balls and place them on a baking sheet lined with parchment paper.
6. Use a fork to press and flatten the dough.

Amount Per Serving

Calories: 109

Fat: 9

Parmesan Crisps

Serves 4

Serving Size: 5 crisps

Ingredients

Parmesan cheese (1 cup)

Coconut flour (4 tablespoons)

Rosemary, oregano or any herbs of choice, dried or fresh (1-2 teaspoons)

Directions

1. Preheat the oven to 350 Fahrenheit. In a small bowl, mix the coconut flour and grated parmesan cheese. Don't use finely grated, or powdery parmesan cheese like you find in a canister at the supermarket, as it won't work well in this recipe. Try to find finely grated parmesan in the deli section of your supermarket, or even better, grate your own!
2. You can add any herbs you like. Oregano and rosemary work wonderfully.
3. Scoop a teaspoon of the cheese mixture onto a baking tray lined with parchment paper leaving a small gap between each. Place in the oven and cook for 10-15 minutes or until golden brown, but be careful not to burn.
4. Remove from the oven and let the crisps cool down before you remove them from the baking tray.
5. Enjoy!

Amount Per Serving

Calories: 233

Fat: 14.5

Mini Pizza Bombs

Serves 6

Ingredients

14 slices Italian sausages

8 pitted black olives

3/4 cup Cream cheese

2 Tbs fresh basil, chopped

2 Tbs pesto

salt and pepper to taste

Directions

1. Dice pitted Kalamata olives and pepperoni into small pieces.
2. Mix together cream cheese, basil and pesto.
3. Add the olives and sausage slices into the cream cheese and mix again.
4. Form into balls and garnish with pepperoni, basil, and olive. Ready!!

Cooking Time: 10 minutes

Nutrition Facts (per serving)

Total Carbohydrates: 3,5g

Dietary Fiber: 0,7g

196

Net Carbs: 1g

Protein: 10,4g

Total Fat: 23,43g

Calories: 261

Cheesy Bacon Fat Bombs

Serves 24

Ingredients

8 strips cooked crispy bacon, crumbled

1 cup cream cheese, softened

1/2 cup butter

4 tsp bacon fat

4 Tbsp coconut oil

1/4 cup Splenda to taste

Directions

1. In a microwave dish, combine all ingredients and melt slowly in the microwave until smooth. Set aside some crumbled bacon,
2. Pour into a dish or pan and place in the freezer until firm, about 30 minutes.
3. Before serving, remove from freezer, sprinkle with more crumbled bacon, slice and serve.

Nutrition Facts (per serving)

Total Carbohydrates: 0,5g

Dietary Fiber: 0g

Net Carbs: 0,3g

Protein: 0g

Total Fat: 15,9g

Calories: 151

Creamy Greek Balls

Serves 5

Ingredients

1 cup cream cheese, softened

1 cup butter, softened

2-3 Tbsp freshly chopped herbs (any combination of basil, thyme, oregano and/or parsley works great) or 2 teaspoons of dried herbs

4 pieces sun-dried tomatoes, drained

4 Kalamata olives, pitted and chopped

2 cloves garlic, crushed

freshly ground black pepper

1 tsp sea salt

5 Tbs parmesan cheese, finely grated

Directions

1. Mash the butter and cream cheese together with a fork and mix until well combined. Mix in the chopped sun-dried tomatoes and chopped Kalamata olives.
2. Add the freshly chopped herbs (or dried), crushed garlic and season with salt and pepper. Mix well and place in the fridge for 20-30 minutes to firm up.
3. Remove the cheese mixture from the fridge and start creating 5 balls. A spoon or an ice-cream scooper works well.

4. Place the grated parmesan cheese in a shallow dish. Roll each ball in the grated parmesan cheese and place on a plate. Eat immediately or store in the fridge in an airtight container for up to a week.
5. Enjoy!

Nutrition Facts (per serving)

Total Carbohydrates: 2,8g

Dietary Fiber: 0,24g

Net Carbs: 0,8g

Protein: 3,67g

Total Fat: 19,8g

Calories: 200

Smoked Turkey, Blue Cheese Eggs

Serves 6

Ingredients

6 eggs

2 green onions

6 oz smoked turkey breast, chopped

1/2 cup blue cheese, crumbled

2 Tbsp Blue cheese dressing

1/4 cup mayonnaise

2 Tbsp hot mustard

1/2 rib celery

Directions

1. Hard boil the eggs, covered for 12 minutes.
2. In a meanwhile, chop up the smoked turkey breast and the celery.
3. Slice eggs in half lengthwise, scrape the yolks out into a bowl. Add the rest of the ingredients (except the green onions).
4. Grate the green onions over the mixture. Mix all ingredients together.
5. With the teaspoon fill every egg with the mixture.
6. Place on a serving plate and refrigerate for one hour. Ready! Serve and enjoy!

Cooking Times

202

Total Time: 20 minutes

Nutrition Facts (per serving)

Total Carbohydrates: 3,9g

Dietary Fiber: 0,3g

Net Carbs: 0,6g

Protein: 14g

Total Fat: 11,5g

Calories: 167

Pancetta & Eggs

Serves 4

Ingredients

4 large slices Pancetta

2 eggs, free-range

1 cup ghee, softened

2 Tbsp mayonnaise

salt and freshly ground black pepper to taste

coconut oil for frying

Directions

1. In a greased non-stick frying pan, bake Pancetta from both side 1-2 minutes. Remove from the fire and set aside.
2. In a meanwhile boil the eggs. To get the eggs hard-boiled, you need round 10 minutes. When done, wash the eggs with cold water well and peel off the shells.
3. In a deep bowl place ghee and add the quartered eggs. Mash with a fork well. Season it with salt and pepper to taste; add mayonnaise and mix. If you want you can pour in the Pancetta grease. Combine and mix well. Place the bowl in the fridge for one hour at least.
4. Remove the egg mixture from the fridge and make 4 equal balls.
5. Crumble the Pancetta into small pieces. Roll each ball in the Pancetta crumbles and place on a big platter.

6. Remove the Egg and Pancetta bombs in a fridge for 30 minutes more. Serve cold.

Nutrition Facts (per serving)

Total Carbohydrates: 2,2g

Dietary Fiber: 0g

Net Carbs: 0,5g

Protein: 7,5g

Total Fat: 22g

Calories: 238

Parmesan, Herb & Sun-dried Tomato Bombs

Serves 4

Ingredients

1 cup cream cheese

1 cup ghee

5 Tbsp parmesan cheese

1/4 cup sun-dried tomatoes, chopped

1/4 cup Kalamata olives, pitted

3 cloves garlic, crushed

3 Tbsp herbs mix (basil, parsley, thyme, oregano, parsnip, mint)

salt and freshly ground black pepper to taste

Directions

1. In a bowl, combine the cream cheese and ghee. Set aside for 30-45 minutes to soft.
2. After, mix the ghee and the cream cheese until well combined. Add the chopped Kalamata olives and sun-dried tomatoes.
3. Add in herbs and crushed garlic; season with salt and pepper to taste. Mix well with the fork and place bowl in the fridge for at least 1 hour.
4. Remove the cheese mixture from the fridge and create 4 balls. Roll each ball in the grated parmesan cheese and place on a plate.
5. Return it to the fridge for 30 minutes. Serve and enjoy.

Cooking Times

Total Time: 1 hour and 20 minutes

Nutrition Facts (per serving)

Total Carbohydrates: 4g

Dietary Fiber: 0,5g

Net Carbs: 1g

Protein: 4,6g

Total Fat: 14g

Calories: 157

Spicy Bacon & Avo Bites

Serves 6

Serving Size: 1 fat bomb

Ingredients

½ large avocado

Butter, softened (1/4 cups)

2 cloves garlic, crushed

Crushed red pepper (1 teaspoon)

½ small white onion, diced

Fresh lime juice (1 tablespoon)

Freshly ground black pepper

Sea salt (¼ teaspoon)

large slices bacon

Bacon grease, reserved from cooking (2 tablespoons)

Directions

1. Preheat the oven to 375 Fahrenheit. Line a baking tray with parchment paper. Lay the bacon strips out flat on the parchment paper, leaving space so they don't overlap. Place the tray in the oven and cook for about 10-15 minutes until golden brown and crisp. The time will depend on the thickness of the bacon slices. When done, remove from the oven and set aside to cool down.

2. Halve, deseed and peel the avocado. Place the avocado, butter, crushed red pepper, crushed garlic and lime juice into a bowl and season with salt and pepper.
3. Mash using a potato masher or a fork until well combined. Add the diced onion and mix well.
4. Pour in the 2 tablespoons of reserved bacon grease and mix well. Cover with foil and place in the fridge for 20-30 minutes to firm up.
5. Chop the bacon into small pieces and place in a shallow dish.
6. Remove the guacamole mixture from the fridge and start creating 6 balls. You can use a spoon or an ice-cream scooper. Roll each ball in the bacon crumbles and place on a tray that will fit in the fridge.
7. Eat immediately or store in the fridge in an airtight container for up to 5 days.

Nutrition Facts (per serving)

Calories: 156

Fat: 15.2

Fried Tuna & Avo Balls

Serves 12

Ingredients

Mayonnaise (1/4 cup)

Parmesan cheese (1/4 cup)

Garlic powder (1/2 teaspoon)

Salt

Canned Tuna (10 oz., drained)

Avocado (1, cubed)

Almond flour (1/3 cup)

Onion powder (1/4 teaspoon)

Coconut oil (1/2 cup)

Directions

1. Combine all ingredients in a bowl except oil and avocado.
2. Add avocado and fold, use hands to form balls and dust with flour.
3. Heat oil in a pot and fry tuna bites until golden all over.
4. Serve.

Nutritional Information per bite

Calories 135

Net Carbs 0.8g

Fats 11.8g

Protein 6.2 g

Fiber 1.2g

Chapter 8

4 Week Keto Meal Plan Sample

Meal Plan – Week One			
	Monday	**Tuesday**	**Wednesday**
Breakfast	*Breakfast Granola*	*Orange Choco-Cashew Smoothie*	*Rosemary, Sausage & Cheese Pies*
Lunch	*Beef Sausage, Bacon & Broccoli Casserole*	*Salmon Salad in Avocado Cups*	Pecorino Romano Breaded Cutlets
Dinner	*Italian Fish Stew*	Spicy Mexican Meatballs	Baked Herb Salmon Fillets
Thursday	**Friday**	**Saturday**	**Sunday**
Easy Pancakes	*Breakfast Berry Shake*	*Mozzarella, Red Pepper & Bacon Frittata*	*Kale Sausage Omelet Pie*
Spicy Chicken Thighs	*Homemade Meatballs*	*Bacon, Lettuce, Tomato Salad*	Chicken & Cauliflower Lasagna

Beef Shin Stew	Keto Burger Patties	Easy, Peasy, Cheese Pizza	Orange Glazed Duck

Meal Plan – Week Two

	Monday	Tuesday	Wednesday
Breakfast	Chia, Coconut & Almond Oatmeal	Egg Pesto Scramble	Cacao and Raspberry Pudding
Lunch	Keto Ham & Grilled Cheese Sandwich	Hearty Salad	Crunchy Chicken Waldorf Salad
Dinner	Pan Fried Hake	Ratatouille	Slow Cookers Oxtail Stew

Thursday	Friday	Saturday	Sunday
Ketogenic Mug Bread	Cream Cheese Pancakes	Breakfast Quiche	Berry Bliss
Broccoli Salad	Bacon, Lettuce, Tomato Salad	Garlic Chicken Thighs	Slow Cooker Chicken Stew
Kale & Chili "Meatballs"	Italian Fish Stew	Chicken Hash	Creamy Haddock

Meal Plan – Week Three

	Monday	Tuesday	Wednesday

214

Breakfast	*Bacon, Scallions & Monterey Omelet*	*Cream Cheese Pancakes*	*Veggie Scramble*
Lunch	*Spring Roll In a Bowl*	*Salmon Salad in Avocado Cups*	*Homemade Meatballs*
Dinner	Almond Bread	*Keto Burger Patties*	*Tuna Fish Stew*

Thursday	**Friday**	**Saturday**	**Sunday**
Breakfast Granola	*Egg Pesto Scramble*	*Lemon Cheesecake Breakfast Mousse*	*Breakfast Quiche*
Cheesy Hotdog Pockets	*Avo & Tuna Lettuce Wraps*	*Zucchini Stuffed with Chicken & Broccoli*	*Savoury Mince*
Bacon, Beef Sausage, and Broccoli Casserole	*Chicken Stir-Fry*	Lamb Cutlets with Garlic Sauce	*Cauliflower Bake*

Meal Plan – Week Four

	Monday	**Tuesday**	**Wednesday**
Breakfast	*Mozzarella, Red Pepper & Bacon*	*Ketogenic Mug Bread*	*Caprese Stack*

	Frittata		+ *Creamy Chocolate Milk*
Lunch	*Beef Shred Salad*	*Spinach Cheese & Bacon Log*	*Greek Salad*
Dinner	*Chicken Parmesan*	*Tender Pork & Bacon Cassoulet*	*Keto Burger Patties*
Thursday	**Friday**	**Saturday**	**Sunday**
Cacao and Raspberry Pudding	*Chia, Coconut & Almond Oatmeal*	*Bacon, Avocado & Smoked Turkey Muffins*	*Breakfast Quiche*
Spicy Chicken Thighs	*Portobello Burgers*	*Warm Chicken Salad*	*Homemade Meatballs*
Creamy Haddock	*Chicken, Bacon & Cream Cheese Pot Pie*	*Lamb Cutlets with Garlic Sauce*	*Slow Cookers Oxtail Stew*

__Conclusion__

Thank you again for purchasing this book!

I hope that you will use what you've learned from this book on your journey to lose weight, and most importantly, become healthier. Yes, there are many diets out there that promises the same results, however, the Ketogenic Diet is one of the few that is scientifically proven that it really works!

Remember, losing weight doesn't mean that you have to skip your meals and starve yourself in order to shed fat. What you just need to do is to watch what you eat—limit your carbs, moderately consume protein, and eat more fat, the healthy type of fat!

The Ketogenic Diet will help you achieve your health goals, but just like any other diets, your commitment and perseverance to follow this diet is needed for you to reap its benefits. Do use the tips, recipes, and meal plans that I shared with you during the first weeks of your Keto Diet. Also, don't be afraid to explore other recipes that you wish to include in your meal plan. As long as you stay within the numbers of the required macros you need to consume, then you're assured that your body is continuously burning fat.

Try the Ketogenic diet and gain mental clarity, burn excess fat and have unlimited energy today.
I wish you great health and good tidings as you set out on this amazing journey to ultimate health.

All the best!

Finally, if you feel that you have received any value from this book, then I'd like to ask if you would be kind enough to click on the link below and leave a review on Amazon to share your positive experience with other

readers.
It'd be greatly appreciated!

permission or backing by the trademark owner. All trademarks and brands within this book are for clarifying purposes only and are the owned by the owners themselves, not affiliated with this document.

The author is not a licensed practitioner, physician or medical professional and offers no medical treatment, diagnoses, suggestions or counseling. The information presented herein has not been evaluated by the U.S Food & Drug Administration, and it is not intended to diagnose, treat, cure or prevent any disease. Full medical clearance from a licensed physician should be obtained before beginning or modifying any diet, exercise or lifestyle program, and physician should be informed of all nutritional changes. The author claims no responsibility to any person or entity for any liability, loss or damage caused or alleged to be caused directly or indirectly as a result of the use, application or interpretation of the information presented herein.

Made in the USA
Middletown, DE
05 July 2016